A Colour Guide to
The Assessment and Management of
LEG ULCERS

2nd Edition

Moya J Morison BSc, MSc, BA, RGN
Postgraduate Research Nurse
Queen Margaret College, Edinburgh

Christine J Moffatt RGN, NDN
Clinical Nurse Specialist Leg Ulcers

M Mosby

Copyright © 1994 Times Mirror International Publishers Limited

Published in 1994 by Mosby, an imprint of Times Mirror International
Publishers Limited

Printed by Grafos S.A. Arte sobre papel, Barcelona, Spain

ISBN 07234 2001 7

First edition published in 1991 by Wolfe Publishing Limited.

For full details of all Times Mirror International Publishers Limited titles,
please write to Times Mirror International Publishers Limited, Lynton
House, 7–12 Tavistock Square, London WC1H 9LB, England

A CIP catalogue record for this book is available from the British Library.

Contents

Foreword

Many nurses will be aware of Moya Morison's previous books on leg ulcers and wound management (1991, 1992). This book, written in conjunction with Christine Moffatt, serves to update that work and to introduce further aspects for consideration in the treatment and care of leg ulcers. It is a pleasure to be asked to write the foreword to this book.

Leg ulcers can be painful, and they are a cause of concern and distress both for those afflicted and for their carers. Consequently, a great deal of Health Service resources, including nursing time, are directed to the care of leg ulcers.

This book lists and discusses the many causes of leg ulcers and emphasises the need for a clear diagnosis of the type of leg ulcer and for the recognition of underlying and concomitant medical conditions. It outlines the need for individualised patient assessment, and this requires appropriate training, education, use of equipment, supervision, and links to vascular services; all of which are aimed at providing a safe and efficient service.

The psychosocial aspects of leg ulcers are considered, and good communication and patient education are highlighted as essential elements of leg ulcer care. The final chapter addresses the very important subjects of quality and audit. It is incumbent on all health care professionals to consider research findings, to reflect on their practice, and where necessary, to adjust in order to provide the most safe, efficient, and cost-effective services.

Those who read this book may wish to be aware that the NHSME included the management of leg ulcers in the Clinical Guidelines Executive letter (21 December, 1993 EL(93), 115) to purchasers.

Mrs Yvonne Moores
Chief Nursing Officer/Director of Nursing
Department of Health
Richmond House
79 Whitehall
London SW1A 2NS

Dedication

To our husbands, Graeme and Stuart, without whose practical help, support and tolerance this book would not have been possible.

Acknowledgements

This book has been made possible by the good will, encouragement and help of many people, including Graeme Morison who proofread the text and helped with the illustrations, and Helen and Alastair Morison who typed the manuscript, and all of its many revisions.

We would also like to thank the following individuals, institutions and organisations who kindly agreed to the use of the following illustrations:

Huntleigh Healthcare: *Figure 32*
Lederle Laboratories: *Figures 36, 37*
Medi (UK): *Figures 31, 33*
Chelsea and Westminster Hospital, Medical Illustrations Department: *Figures 14, 15*
Perstorp Pharma: *Figures 39, 40*
Charing Cross Hospital, Regional Vascular Service: *Figures 7, 10, 16, 17, 20, 21, 41; Appendices 5.2, 5.3*
Bloom, A. and Ireland, J. (1992) *A Colour Atlas of Diabetes* (2nd edn) Wolfe Publishing: *Figures 11, 12, 13*
Farthing C. F., Brown, S. E. and Staughton, R. C. D. (1988) *A Colour Atlas of AIDS and HIV Disease* (2nd edn) Wolfe Medical Publications: *Figures 18, 19*
Ruckley, C. V. (1988) *A Colour Atlas of Surgical Management of Venous Disease* Wolfe Publishing: *Figures 9, 22, 34, 38*
Stone, L. A., Lindfield, E. M. and Robertson, S. (1989) *A Colour Atlas of Nursing Procedures in Skin Disorders* Wolfe Medical Publications Ltd. *Figure 28*

1. Epidemiology, service provision and health economics

1.0 Introduction

This chapter sets the scene for the chapters which follow by reviewing the epidemiology of leg ulcers, describing who routinely carries out their care, and summarising what is known about the cost of leg ulcers, both for the individual and for the NHS.

Epidemiology is the study of the distribution of a disease or a pathophysiological condition in human populations and the factors that influence this distribution (Lilienfeld, 1978). Epidemiologists seek answers to a number of questions. How common is a condition? Is it becoming more or less common? Who is most at risk? This information is necessary to inform the planning of a service (Chapter 7) and to help to target primary and secondary prevention programmes to the highest risk groups (Section 4.1.8). It can also give clues about the underlying causes of a condition (Chapter 2).

The commonness of a condition can be expressed in terms of its incidence or its prevalence. *Incidence* is the proportion of *new* cases in the population that occur during a given time period. *Prevalence* is the proportion of the population at a *particular point in time* with the condition.

Most of the studies of the epidemiology of leg ulcers have measured prevalence. Their relatively high prevalence, compared to their incidence, is a reflection of their slow healing and high recurrence rates.

The dramatic effects of community clinics in improving healing rates and reducing costs are outlined in Sections 1.4 and 1.5 and demonstrate how much can be achieved in a relatively short time when 'best practice' principles are consistently applied.

The purpose of this book is to describe best practice and the underlying principles, derived from the latest clinical research. The authors aim to give a balanced review of a variety of treatment options available and emphasise the paramount importance of accurate and ongoing patient assessment (Chapter 3).

1.1 The size of the problem

Large scale studies both in the UK and in mainland Europe, suggest that 1–2% of the population develop a leg ulcer at some point in their lives (Laing, 1992). About one fifth of these people have an open ulcer at any one time (Callam *et al.*, 1985). The problem of leg ulceration rises markedly with age, particularly for those in their 70s and 80s. In less developed countries those aged 65 and over account for 5% or less of the total population, but in Britain the proportion of the total population aged 65 and over now exceeds 15% (Grundy, 1992). While the projected increases in the relative size of the elderly population in the next 20 years are fairly slight for the UK, the size of the 80+ age group is set to grow significantly (Rose, 1993). This is a major cause for concern with obvious health economic implications. Venous ulcers in which there is an arterial component are most common in this age group and are a very difficult type to treat.

Under the age of 40 the prevalence of ulceration in men and women is similar, but with increasing age the prevalence in women is higher. The reasons for this gender difference are unclear. Leg ulceration is often regarded as a problem of old age, but when analysing the age at onset of the first episode of ulceration, Callam *et al.* (1987) found that more than one third of patients had ulcers before they were 50 and more than two thirds before the age of 65.

The recurrence rate for ulceration is also depressing, with about two thirds of patients experiencing two or more episodes and 21% of patients more than six episodes. There is an old adage: 'Once an ulcer patient, always a potential ulcer patient'. This is borne out by a survey which showed that half the patients with an ulcer had a history of ulceration dating back at least ten years.

1.2   Risk factors for ulceration

It was once thought that leg ulcers were mainly associated with low socio-economic status, but this was not borne out by a study by Callam *et al.* (1988). This study did, however, show that when leg ulceration occurred it was more likely to be recurrent and to take longer to heal in the more disadvantaged socio-economic groups.

Venous insufficiency and varicose veins are more common in patients with venous ulcers than without, but it is not clear whether these are associated conditions with a common aetiology or predisposing factors for ulcers (Fletcher, 1991). Deep vein thrombosis (DVT) has frequently been cited as the predisposing factor to chronic venous hypertension and venous ulceration (Section 2.1). The problem is that many people suffer from DVT without being aware of it. Even for those people with leg ulcers, for whom a previous history of DVT has been unequivocally established, correlation does not prove causation. There is a great deal to be learned about risk factors for leg ulcers.

A recent study suggests that reduced general mobility and reduced limb mobility are significant risk factors. They are certainly common problems, associated with increasing age and with delayed ulcer healing (Section 1.4). Risk factors for venous disease are reviewed by Moffatt and Franks (1994).

1.3   Who carries out the care?

Over 80% of all leg ulcer patients are cared for in the community by district and practice nurses, or by relatives who may or may not be adequately instructed or supervised (Cornwall *et al.*, 1986). Many patients have never been referred for a specialist opinion, although their ulcers may have been open for many years (Lees and Lambert, 1992).

Those who are referred to hospital outpatient clinics may be seen by a variety of specialists including dermatologists, vascular surgeons and physicians with a special interest in wound healing. While there are many centres of excellence, overall provision of specialist care and the organisation of an integrated hospital and community leg ulcer service is patchy in the UK (Gilliland and Wolfe, 1991).

Recent studies of leg ulcer management have shown that dramatic improvements in healing rates can be achieved when services are rationalised and research-based protocols are consistently implemented (Moffatt *et al.*, 1992) (Section 1.4). *Table 1* illustrates how healing rates improved with time after setting up each new Community Clinic in the Riverside project. This occurred because patients were referred earlier and the chronic, long-standing ulcers were progressively healed.

Only a very small percentage of patients with leg ulcers receive treatment in hospital on an inpatient basis. The main reasons for planned admission are:

- For skin grafting.
- For a comprehensive vascular assessment.
- For vascular surgery.
- To reduce gross oedema where all other methods have failed.
- To control pain.

For some patients, the ulcer is not the primary reason for admission, but is noticed and treated 'in passing'. Individuals may remain in hospital for protracted periods, at a high financial and personal cost.

Table 1. Healing rates of all patients with leg ulceration, to 12 weeks of treatment, by time of referral after start of each clinic (compared with control study) (based on Moffatt et al, 1992, p. 1391)

Time of referral after setting up of each new clinic	Cumulative percentage healed
15–18 months	86
6–9 months	78
0–3 months	55
Control	22

1.4   Treatment times and healing rates

Leg ulcers are notoriously slow to heal. In one study, 50% of ulcers had been open for one year or more (Cornwall *et al.*, 1986). In another study, 50% of patients with current ulcers reported that the ulcer had been open for up to 9 months, 20% had not healed after two years, and 8% were still open after 5 years (Callam *et al.*, 1987).

In a recent audit study of the wound care carried out by community nurses, 22% of their patients had had an open ulcer for 1–5 years, and 6% for more than 5 years (Morison, 1992). Although in this study leg ulcers represented only 21.6%, or 127 of the 589 wounds being treated during the study week, these patients had, overall, undergone treatment for far longer than patients with other open wounds such as pressure sores, sinuses and abscesses, and for very much longer than patients with traumatic or surgically made wounds (*Figure 1*).

The longest reported duration of a single episode of ulceration in Callam *et al.*'s 1987 study was 62 years in an 85 year old lady who had been kicked by a cow while working as a milkmaid during the First World War. Chronic leg ulceration may plague some people for virtually the whole of their adult life.

Some of the factors which affect healing rates include the ulcer's underlying aetiology, ulcer area, the duration of ulceration and the age of the patient (Skene *et al.*, 1992). Cumulative healing rates from the Riverside Community Clinic's study are illustrated in *Table 2*. In this study the duration of the ulcer prior to the patient's first attendance at the clinic was found to be very important. Cumulative healing rates at 24 weeks from commencement of treatment were found to be 91% in ulcers which had been open for up to 6 months prior to treatment, compared with only 72% for leg ulcers of more than 6 months' duration. This has very important implications for practice. It confirms the universally accepted and self evident principle that the sooner a patient receives *appropriate* care, the better the prognosis.

A corollary to this is of relevance to managers, purchasers of services, and to researchers conducting clinical trials of treatment methods. It can be very misleading to compare healing rates between centres in different parts of Britain unless the characteristics of the patient population that they treat are the same. The availability of specialist services, referral patterns and referral criteria vary widely throughout the UK. A service to which in general only the 'worst case', intractable ulcers are referred is almost inevitably going to have worse healing rates than a new or relatively new service which takes all-comers, if this includes a high proportion of patients whose ulcers have been open for less than 6 months (*Table 2*). Each may be providing an equally competent service. It would also be quite unjust to castigate staff for poor healing rates if they have quickly healed the newest ulcers in their catchment area, and are left to manage a caseload of patients with largely intractable ulcers.

To what extent is delayed ulcer healing with increasing age due to a reduction in the healing capacity of the skin itself? The three phases of healing – inflammation, proliferation and remodelling – still occur,

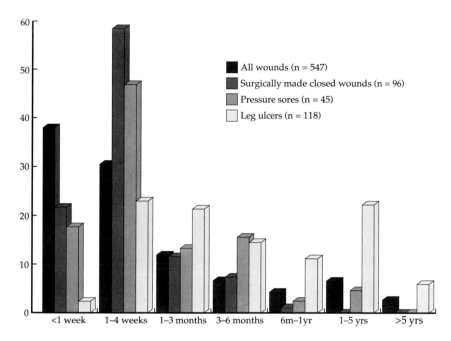

Figure 1 Length of time that wounds have been treated in the community (% of wounds in each category). (Based on Morison, 1992)

Table 2. Some factors affecting cumulative healing rates for venous ulcers at 12 and 24 weeks from commencement of treatment (based on Moffatt *et al.*, 1992, p. 1391)

Factor	Number of cases	Cumulative Percentage Healed	
		12 weeks	24 weeks
• Ulcer Area			
< 10 cm^2	336	80	92
≥ 10 cm^2	128	42	61
• Duration of ulcer			
< 1 month	178	74	90
1–6 months	93	80	92
> 6 months	186	57	72
• Mobility			
Walking freely	235	73	86
Walking with aid	148	71	84
Bed- or chair-bound	28	48	70

although they may be slower in the elderly (Eaglestein, 1989). Reduced activity of macrophages with increasing age has been implicated. However, there seem to be sufficient reserves in the healing processes to allow effective and complete healing even into very old age. The effects of ageing on skin and skin related disorders are extensively reviewed by Dalziel and Bickers (1992) and Mast (1992).

5

1.5 The financial cost of leg ulceration and venous disease

In the UK, recently reported estimates of the costs of managing leg ulcers have ranged from £150–600 million per annum. The upper end of this range is almost certainly an overestimate. As part of a European study of the cost of venous disease, the Office of Health Economics estimated the cost in the UK of venous disease of the legs, including the cost of varicose vein management and costs associated with venous insufficiency, phlebitis, and thrombophlebitis, to have been £294 million in 1989 (Laing, 1992). This is 2% of total health care spending in the UK. A high proportion of this is estimated to have been the cost of District Nursing services.

In a recent study of District Nursing grades and skill mix in relation to workload, it was found that the principal purpose of 29.2% of visits was wound care, 44.7% of which (or 13.06% of the total visits) were specifically for the management of leg ulcers. Wound care figured prominently in the top ten purposes of visits, which accounted for 70% of the total (NHS Management Executive Value for Money Unit, 1992).

Estimates of the actual time spent by community nurses in treating patients with leg ulcers vary from 10–50%. One survey in an urban Health District found that 7% of patients with ulcers were having their dressings changed daily, 28% three times a week, 35% twice a week, 27% once a week, and 3% less than once a week (Lees and Lambert, 1992). The average treatment time per visit (excluding travelling time) was 23 minutes. Similar results were found in a more general audit of wound care in the community (*Table 3*). In this study the average number of nurse/patient contacts per week for leg ulcer management was 2, ranging from daily to weekly (Morison, 1992).

More detailed data on treatment costs has come from the Riverside project. For patients with ulcers treated continuously over a two year period treatment costs were £1067 per patient per annum. Treatment costs for all patients were £670 per patient (Bosanquet, 1992). These costs included the costs of bandages, district nurse time, outpatient and inpatient visits, general practitioner consultations and prescribing.

Healing rates vary very widely between and within Health Authorities. The changes in the health service arising from the Government's White Paper 'Working for Patients' are encouraging the development of programmes which are both beneficial to patients and cost-effective and efficient, for instance through the introduction of purchasing contracts which require that providers develop programmes with defined aims and standards of care (Teasdale, 1992).

An evaluation of a range of different organisational models is required. Outpatient clinics run by clinicians with a strong interest in the management of leg ulceration can achieve excellent results, but the difficulty lies in replicating the high quality of service (Laing, 1992). In the community where most patients with leg ulcers are managed, the challenge is to ensure that nurses have the requisite skills for the assessment and management of routine cases and know when to refer patients on for more specialist assessment. The Riverside project demonstrated that by investing time and resources in an innovative community programme linked to a vascular service, the cost of caring could be reduced in the long term (Bosanquet, 1992; Bosanquet et al., 1994). This model is described in Chapter 7.

It is estimated that by the year 2000, there will be an increase of 43% in the very elderly aged over 85. This group has the highest leg ulcer prevalence. If current demographic trends continue demands for leg ulcer treatment are likely to rise rather than fall, which gives further impetus to the need to develop 'best practice' guidelines. Furthermore, patients' attitudes and expectations may change. Future generations may be less tolerant of chronic disabling conditions such as leg ulceration. The demand for more effective treatment may increasingly come from *patients* as well as from professionals (Bosanquet, 1992).

Table 3. Time to assess and dress wounds in the community (based on Morison, 1992)

Type of wound	Number of cases	Mean time to assess and dress wounds (min/week)
Minor traumatic wounds	154	17.2
Leg ulcers	127	31.9
Surgically made, closed wounds	104	22.5
Minor non-traumatic wounds	65	21.2
Pressure sores	53	22.9
Diabetic foot ulcers	25	38.1
Sinuses	24	40.4
Abcesses	16	32.7

1.6   Impact of leg ulcers on quality of life

What impact does a leg ulcer have on the quality of a person's life?

There have been several studies on the influence of cardiovascular disease and its treatment on quality of life. These include Drory and Florian's 1991 study of long term psychosocial adjustment to coronary artery disease, Daumer and Miller's 1990 study of the effects of cardiac rehabilitation on psychosocial functioning and life satisfaction, and Hunt et al.'s 1982 study of the subjective health of people with peripheral vascular disease, using the Nottingham Health Profile. However, there is a paucity of data specific to patients with leg ulcers.

In a study of the socio-economic aspects of chronic leg ulceration Callam et al. (1988) found that the condition interfered with work or leisure activities to a moderate or severe degree in 42% of patients, although in only 11% of patients was mobility affected by leg ulceration alone. In a study of patient's perceptions of chronic leg ulceration, over a third of patients felt that the worst thing about having an ulcer was the pain associated with it (Hamer et al., 1993)

A symptom rating test carried out among patients prior to and after 12 weeks of treatment using the four-layer bandage method developed at

Charing Cross Hospital demonstrated improved quality of life with significant reduction in depression, anxiety and hostility, and improved cognitive function (Franks *et al.*, 1994). In a long term follow-up study of patients with venous ulceration, 42% of patients with healed ulcers reported improved mobility, 10% improvements in sleep and 18% a reduction in pain. Of those with an unhealed ulcer, 33% had nevertheless experienced a general improvement in health and 28% a reduction in pain.

Cox *et al.* (1992), Fitzpatrick *et al.* (1992) and Fletcher *et al.* (1992) have reviewed issues and practicalities relating to the assessment of quality of life as applied to health care. Spiegelhalter *et al.* (1992) and Hopkins (1992) discuss the controversial issue of quality adjusted life years in relation to resource allocation. The effects of ulcer healing on quality of life are reviewed by Franks *et al.* (1994).

It is becoming increasingly evident that leg ulcers do have a significant impact on patients' quality of life. The importance of quality of life as an outcome measure when auditing leg ulcer care is discussed further in Chapter 6, which looks in more detail at quality assurance.

References

Bosanquet, N. (1992) Cost of venous ulcers: from maintenance therapy to investment programmes. *Phlebology* Supplement 1, 44-46.

Bosanquet, N., Franks, P.J., Moffatt, C.J., Connolly, M.J., Oldroyd, M.I., Brown, P., Greenhalgh, R.M. & McCollum, C.N. (1994) Community leg ulcer clinics: cost effectiveness. *Health Trends* **(in press)**.

Callam, M.J., Harper, D.R., Dale, J.J. & Ruckley, C.V. (1987) Chronic ulcer of the leg: clinical history. *BMJ* **294**, 1389-1391.

Callam, M.J., Harper, D.R., Dale, J.J. & Ruckley, C.V. (1988) Chronic leg ulceration: socio-economic aspects. *Scott Med J* **33**, 358-360.

Callam, M.J., Ruckley, C.V., Harper, D.R. & Dale, J.J. (1985) Chronic ulceration of the leg: extent of the problem and provision of care. *BMJ* **290**, 1855-1856.

Cornwall, J., Dore, C.J. & Lewis, J.D. (1986) Leg ulcers: epidemiology and aetiology. *Br J Surg* **73**, 693-696.

Cox, D., Fitzpatrick, R., Fletcher, A., Gore, S., Spiegelhalter, D. & Jones, D. (1992) Quality of life assessment: can we keep it simple? *Journal of the Royal Statistical Society Series A* **155**, 353-393.

Dalziel, K.L. & Bickers, D.R. (1992) Skin aging. In: Brocklehurst, J.C., Tallis, R.C. & Fillit, H.M. (eds) *Textbook of Geriatric Medicine and Gerontology*, (4th edn), Churchill Livingstone, Edinburgh, pp. 898-921.

Daumer, R. & Miller, P. (1990) Effects of cardiac rehabilitation on psychosocial functioning and life satisfaction of coronary artery disease clients. *Rehabilitation Nursing* **17(2)**, 69-75, 86.

Drory, Y. & Florian, V. (1991) Long-term psychosocial adjustment to coronary artery disease. *Arch Phys Med Rehabil* **72(5)**, 326-331.

Eaglestein, W.H. (1989) Wound healing and aging. *Clin Geriatr Med* **5(1)**, 183-188.

Fitzpatrick, R., Fletcher, A., Gore, S., Jones, D., Spiegelhalter, D. & Cox, D. (1992) Quality of life measures in health care. I: Applications and issues in assessment. *BMJ* **305**, 1074-1077.

Fletcher, A. (1991) Venous ulcers: occurrence and risk factors. *Wound Management* **1(1)**, 11–12.

Fletcher, A., Gore, S., Jones, D., Fitzpatrick, R., Spiegelhalter, D. & Cox, D. (1992) Quality of life measures in health care II: Design, analysis, and interpretation. *BMJ* **305**, 1145–1148.

Franks, P.J., Moffatt, C.J., Connolly, M.J., Bosanquet, N., Oldroyd, M., Greenhalgh, R.M. & McCollum, C.N. (1994) Community leg ulcer clinics: effect on quality of life. *Phlebology* **(in press)**.

Gilliland, E.L. & Wolfe, J.H.N. (1991) Leg ulcers. *BMJ* **303**, 776–779.

Grundy, E. (1992) The epidemiology of aging. In: Brocklehurst, J.C., Tallis, J.C. & Fillit, H.M. (eds) *Textbook of Geriatric Medicine and Gerontology* (4th edn) Churchill Livingstone, Edinburgh, pp. 3–20.

Hamer, C., Cullum, N.A., & Roe, B.H. (1993) Patients' perceptions of chronic leg ulceration. In: Harding, K.G. *et al.* (eds) Proceedings of the 2nd European Conference on advances in wound management, Harrogate 1992. Macmillan Magazines, London, pp. 178–180.

Hopkins, A. (ed) (1992) *Measures of the quality of life: and the uses to which such measures may be put* Royal College of Physicians, London.

Hunt, S. *et al.*, (1982) Subjective health of patients with peripheral vascular disease. *The Practitioner* **226**, 133–136.

Laing, W. (1992) *Chronic venous diseases of the leg* Office of Health Economics, London.

Lees, T.A & Lambert, D., (1992) Prevalence of lower limb ulceration in an urban health district. *Br J Surg* **79**, 1032–1034.

Lilienfeld, D.E. (1978) Definitions of epidemiology. *Am J Epidemiol* **107**, 87–90.

Mast, B.A. (1992) The skin. In: Cohen, I.K., Diegelmann, R.F. & Lindblad, W.J. (eds) *Wound healing: biochemical and clinical aspects* WB Saunders, Philadelphia, pp. 344–355.

Moffatt, C., Franks, P.J., Oldroyd, M., Bosanquet, N., Brown, P., Greenhalgh, R.M. & McCollum, C.N. (1992) Community Clinics for leg ulcers and impact on healing. *BMJ* **305**, 1389–1392.

Moffatt, C.J. & Franks, P.J. (1994) Venous disease risk factors: a review of the evidence. *Professional Nurse* **(in press)**.

Morison, M.J. (1992) Quality assurance and wound care in the community. *Ostomy/Wound Management* **38(8)**, 38–44.

NHS Management Executive Value for Money Unit, (1992) *The nursing skillmix in the District Nursing Service* HMSO, London.

Rose, P. (ed) (1993) *Social Trends 23 (1993 Edition)* Central Statistical Office, HMSO, London.

Skene, A.I., Smith, J.M., Dore, C.J., Charlett, A. & Lewis, J.D. (1992) Venous ulcers: a prognostic index to predict time to healing. *BMJ* **305**, 1119–1121.

Spiegelhalter, D.J., Gore, S.M., Fitzpatrick, R., Fletcher, A.E., Jones, D.R. & Cox, D.R. (1992) Quality of life measures in healthcare. III: Resource allocation. *BMJ* **305**, 1205–1209.

Teasdale, K. (ed) (1992) *Managing the changes in health care: an explanation and exploration of the implications for the NHS of Working for Patients* Wolfe, London.

2 Causes of leg ulcers

2.0 Introduction

A number of pathological conditions are associated with lower limb ulceration, some acting through more than one mechanism (*Table 4*). While a minor traumatic incident is usually the immediate cause of the ulcer, the underlying problem is usually vascular in the UK, western Europe and the USA. In less developed countries the commonest causes of ulceration are trauma and infection (Landra, 1988).

In the UK over 70% of leg ulcers are primarily the result of *chronic venous hypertension* (Section 2.1). *Poor arterial blood supply* accounts for about 10% of leg ulcers (Section 2.2), and a further 10–15% of ulcers are of *mixed arterial and venous origin*. Problems with peripheral arterial circulation involving small or large blood vessels are commonly encountered in patients with rheumatoid arthritis (Section 2.3), and diabetes mellitus (Section 2.4). Arterial problems can be overlooked when the patient also displays the classic signs of chronic venous hypertension in the lower limb.

Table 4. Causes of leg ulcers

1. Principal causes

    - *Chronic venous hypertension,* usually due to incompetent valves in the deep and perforating veins.
    - *Arterial disease* e.g. atherosclerotic occlusion of large vessels leading to tissue ischaemia.
    - Combined chronic venous hypertension and arterial disease.

2. More unusual causes (2–5% in total).

    - *Neuropathy* e.g. associated with diabetes mellitus, spina bifida, leprosy.
    - *Vasculitis* e.g. associated with rheumatoid arthritis, polyarteritis nodosum.
    - *Malignancy* e.g. squamous cell carcinoma, melanoma, basal cell carcinoma, Kaposi's sarcoma.
    - *Infection* e.g. tuberculosis, leprosy, syphilis, fungal infections.
    - *Blood disorders* e.g. polycythaemia, sickle cell disease, thalassaemia.
    - *Metabolic disorder* e.g. pyoderma gangrenosum, pretibial myxoedema.
    - *Lymphoedema.*
    - *Trauma* e.g. lacerations, burns, irradiation injuries.
    - *Iatrogenic* e.g. over-tight bandaging, ill-fitting plaster cast.
    - *Self-inflicted.*

More unusual causes of ulceration, amounting to no more than 2–5% of the total, include malignancy, infection, lymphoedema, blood disorders, and certain metabolic disorders (Section 2.5). A few leg ulcers are primarily due to trauma, some are a secondary complication of treatment, and an unknown proportion are self-inflicted.

Understanding the aetiology of leg ulcers is a prerequisite to systematic and sound clinical assessment, and to planning the most appropriate care. At best, failure to identify and treat the underlying cause of the ulcer can lead to an avoidable delay in healing. At worst, inadequate patient assessment and inappropriate treatment can precipitate the need to amputate the limb.

2.1   Venous ulcers

An understanding of the cause of venous ulceration requires an understanding of the anatomy of the venous system of the lower limb and the mechanics of its blood flow.

2.1.1   Anatomy of the venous system and mechanics of blood flow

Both superficial and deep systems of veins are found in the leg (*Figure 2*). The superficial long and short saphenous veins are designed to carry blood under low pressure, and have many valves to prevent back flow. They lie outside the deep fascia and drain into the deep venous system, which comprises the popliteal and femoral veins. The deep veins are designed to carry blood back to the heart under much higher pressure, and they have fewer valves. The superficial and deep systems are connected by perforating veins which pass through the fascia. Blood is returned to the heart from the periphery, via the venous system, by a combination of mechanisms acting together; these include compression of the veins by muscle contraction, and variations in intra-abdominal and intrathoracic pressure.

Active calf muscles, in their semirigid fascial envelope, act as a pump, forcing deep venous blood upwards towards the heart. When healthy and intact, the valves in the perforating veins prevent back flow of blood to the superficial system (*Figure 3*). During periods of muscle relaxation, blood flows from the superficial veins to an area of temporarily lower pressure in the deep veins (beneath the closed valves), filling them, before the calf muscle pump acts again to force this blood centrally away from the extremities. If the valves in the perforating veins become incompetent (*Figure 4*), the back pressure is transmitted directly to the superficial venous system, reversing the flow, damaging more distal valves, and eventually leading to varicose veins. Damaged valves in the deep and perforating veins are one cause of *chronic venous hypertension* in the lower limb, the high back pressure causing *venous stasis* and *oedema*.

The ankle movement involved in walking is also important, as tensioning and relaxing the Achilles tendon alternately stretches and relaxes the calf muscle independently of calf muscle contraction, further aiding venous return. Emptying of the foot veins is facilitated by external pressure as the heel strikes the ground during walking (Gardner and Fox,

1986). In patients who are 'off their feet', neither the foot pump nor the calf muscle pump can operate, and the efficiency of venous return is markedly impaired.

Some patients' mobility is limited by restricted ankle movement, as seen in people with, for example, extensive ulceration in the gaiter area, lipodermatosclerosis (hardening of the dermis and underlying subcutaneous fat) or with extensive fibrosis. Restricted ankle movement makes venous return of blood to the heart much less efficient.

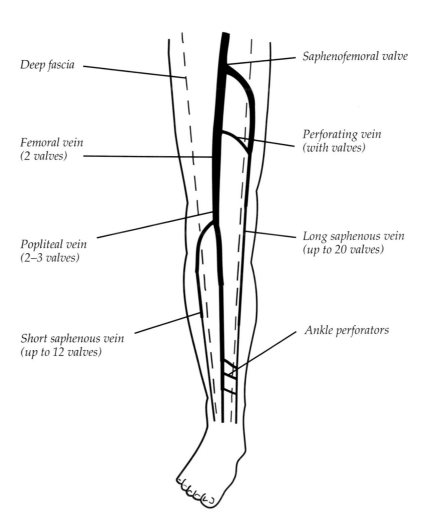

Figure 2. A diagrammatic representation of the normal anatomy of the venous system of the leg (based on Orr and McAvoy, 1987). (For anatomical illustration see, for example, Negus, 1991, or Seeley et al., 1992.)

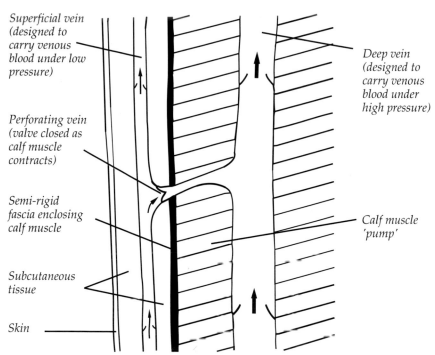

Superficial vein (designed to carry venous blood under low pressure)

Deep vein (designed to carry venous blood under high pressure)

Perforating vein (valve closed as calf muscle contracts)

Semi-rigid fascia enclosing calf muscle

Calf muscle 'pump'

Subcutaneous tissue

Skin

Figure 3. Healthy, intact valves prevent backflow of blood from the deep to the superficial veins.

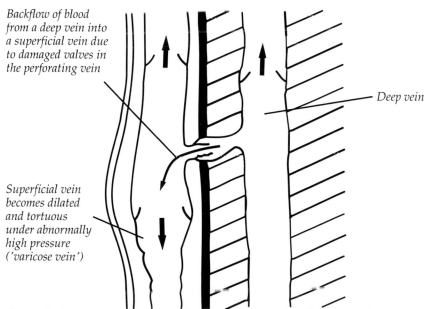

Backflow of blood from a deep vein into a superficial vein due to damaged valves in the perforating vein

Deep vein

Superficial vein becomes dilated and tortuous under abnormally high pressure ('varicose vein')

Figure 4. An incompetent valve in a perforating vein allows backflow of blood from the deep to the superficial venous system.

2.1.2   Clinical signs of chronic venous hypertension

Some of the complications arising from chronic venous hypertension, including varicose veins, stasis eczema and lipodermatosclerosis are summarised in *Figure 5* and described below.

Varicose veins Varicose veins are a common problem, found in 10–20% of the adult population. People in occupations which involve prolonged standing in warm conditions, such as nurses, teachers and warehousemen, are particularly at risk (*Table 5*).

Varicose veins are a sign of chronic venous hypertension in the lower limb, which is usually due to damage to the valves in the leg veins. The damage may be congenital or acquired (*Table 6*). The result is that the superficial venous network is exposed to much higher pressures than normal (up to 90 mmHg instead of 30 mmHg). The superficial veins, especially the relatively thin-walled tributaries of the long and short saphenous veins, become dilated, lengthened and tortuous. About 3% of patients with varicose veins go on to develop leg ulcers but not all patients with venous ulcers have varicose veins. It is therefore not clear whether varicose veins and venous ulcers are merely associated conditions with a common aetiology, or whether varicose veins are a predisposing factor for venous ulcers.

Table 5. Factors thought to predispose the development of varicose veins

- *Family history.*
- *Occupation:* those involving standing in warm conditions.
- *Gender:* more common in women than men with increasing age.
- *Pregnancy.*
- *Low fibre diet.*
- *Obesity.*

Table 6. Causes of varicose veins and raised venous pressure in the lower leg

1.   Primary

- Due to congenital defect in the vein wall (e.g. collagen defect).
- Due to valve cusps absent or abnormal.

2.   Secondary

- *Obstructed venous return* due to pregnancy, pelvic tumours or ascites; can lead to prolonged back pressure in the venous system and incompetent deep and perforating vein valves.
- *Distortion of the valve cusps* caused by deep vein thrombosis, resulting, for example, from leg injury, prolonged immobility, pregnancy or surgery.

Staining of skin in the gaiter area Chronic venous hypertension leads to distension of the blood capillaries, with resulting damage to the endothelial walls, and leakage of red blood cells and large protein molecules into the interstitial fluid (*Figure 5*). Destruction of the red blood

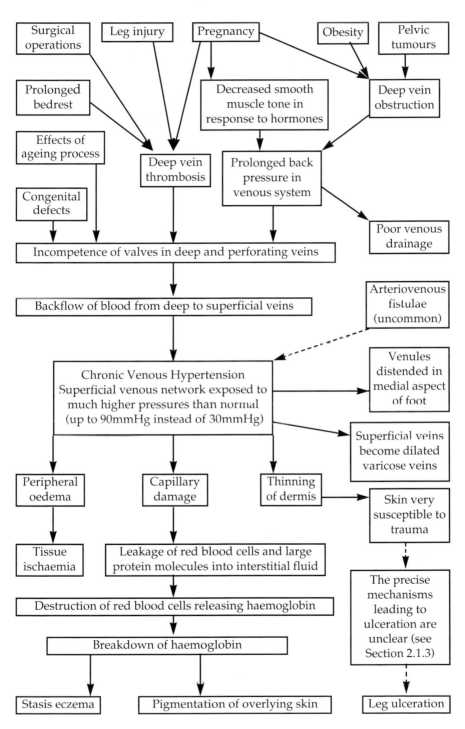

Figure 5. Complications arising from chronic venous hypertension.

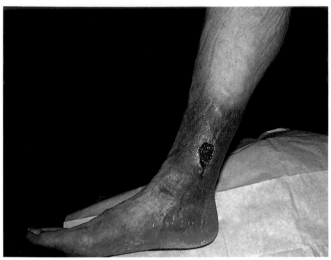

Figure 6. A venous ulcer.

cells releases breakdown products of haemoglobin, leading to pigmentation of the overlying skin (*Figure 6*).

Ankle flare Chronic venous hypertension can cause distension of the tiny veins on the medial aspect of the foot. This is particularly noticeable where the valves in the perforating veins in the ankle and lower calf are incompetent, and is sometimes referred to as 'ankle flare'.

Atrophy of the skin Thinning of the dermis, associated with a poor blood supply, makes the skin very susceptible to trauma. Other trophic changes include stasis eczema and lipodermatosclerosis.

Eczema Eczematous changes to the skin are often associated with venous insufficiency and can be aggravated by a number of wound care products through irritation and allergy (Section 4.6.2.6).

Lipodermatosclerosis 'Woody' induration of the tissues and fat replacement by fibrosis is seen as an end-stage phenomenon. The leg often assumes the shape of an 'inverted champagne bottle', wide at the knee and very narrow at the ankle.

2.1.3   Theories of the cause of venous ulcers

The risk factors for venous ulceration were briefly described in Section 1.2. However, the precise mechanisms leading to ulceration are still the subject of intense debate. Two main theories have emerged.

2.1.3.1 The fibrin cuff theory From biopsy specimens taken from the ulcer bearing skin of 41 legs of 21 patients attending the varicose vein clinic, Burnand *et al.* (1982) demonstrated the presence of layers of fibrin laid down as cuffs around the dermal capillaries in all 26 legs of patients with lipodermatosclerosis. None of the specimens from the legs of 15 patients with clinically normal skin contained fibrin. Browse and Burnand (1982) proposed that as a result of venous hypertension, large molecules, such as fibrinogen, leak out through enlarged pores of damaged and distended dermal blood vessels, and are rapidly polymerised to fibrin. They suggested that these fibrin cuffs form a barrier to the passage of oxygen and other nutrients, which sustain the cells of the epidermis, leading directly to cell death and ulceration. They suggested that, at an early stage, the process could be reversed by reducing venous pressure through surgery or the use of elastic graduated compression stockings, and by enhancing the fibrinolytic activity of the cells with drugs. However, they proposed that, in time, the unchecked deposition of fibrin results in irreversible fibrosis and permanent tissue damage, leading to intractable ulceration, resistant to all currently available treatment.

In a more recent study of the sequential changes in histology and extracellular matrix deposition during the healing of chronic venous ulcers, Herrick *et al.* (1992) have found that these fibrin cuffs contain many other substances, such as laminin, fibronectin and collagen. Thus, the cuffs are not formed purely by the accumulation of blood-borne products extravasated through the vessel walls, but are actively assembled by the adjacent connective tissue cells, in response to increased venous pressure. These cuffs may protect the delicate vessels and enable them to withstand the higher pressures. They demonstrated, histologically, that these fibrin cuffs lyse during healing and eventually disappear.

2.1.3.2 The white cell trapping theory Thomas *et al.* (1988) demonstrated that white cells accumulate in the dependent legs of patients with venous hypertension, and proposed that the trophic skin changes typically seen in patients with venous hypertension (Section 2.1.2) may be aggravated by damage caused by the repeated accumulation of white cells in the microcirculation. Coleridge Smith *et al.* (1988) suggested that the trapped cells become activated, and release toxic metabolites and proteolytic enzymes that result in both damage to, and increased permeability of, the capillaries. Occlusion of capillaries with leukocytes could result in local ischaemia and ulceration.

2.1.3.3 A combination of mechanisms? Herrick *et al.* (1992) suggest that the two apparently divergent hypotheses of venous ulceration, namely the fibrin cuff theory and the white cell trapping theory, are describing different aspects of a sequence of events. They suggest that trapped white cells release a cocktail of cytokines (substances produced by cells as local messengers to other cells) which result in the synthesis of complex vessel 'cuffs'. These inhibit angiogenesis (new blood vessel formation), and nutrient and oxygen diffusion and perfusion, so perpetuating the tissue damage. They propose that as venous return is improved by compression, white cell trapping is reduced, cytokine levels fall and the cuffs are no longer synthesised, but degraded. They observed that disappearing vascular cuffs correlate with epithelialisation, and are predictive of the stage of ulcer healing.

Dalziel and Bickers (1992) concur that all of the events described in these theories probably contribute to skin ischaemia and ulceration. However, they suggest that whatever the changes in the *microcirculation*, these are secondary in importance to abnormalities in the *main venous drainage system* of the lower leg, and in particular to abnormalities in the deep venous system (Section 2.1.1), which are often accompanied by incompetent perforating veins (*Figure 4*).

The mainstay of venous ulcer management, namely graduated compression of the lower limb, aims to reduce the pressures within the superficial venous system, aid venous return of blood to the heart via the deep venous system, and to reduce local oedema (Section 4.1). The contribution of pharmacological agents, which may act at the microcirculatory level, is referred to in Section 4.6.5.

2.2 Arterial ulcers

Arterial ulcers are caused by an insufficient arterial blood supply to the lower limb, resulting in tissue ischaemia and necrosis (*Figure 7*). Occlusion may occur in major or more distal arteries, and may be chronic or acute (*Table 7*).

Atherosclerosis is by far the commonest cause, and is the deposition and accumulation of fatty material in the walls of arteries to form plaques. The process begins before the age of 10 years, being seen then as lipid streaks. It begins to be clinically significant in the teenage years. As well as leading to the narrowing of the lumen of the vessels, causing increased resistance to blood flow and more work for the heart, the plaques increasingly cause fissures and haemorrhages, which in turn may lead to thrombosis, embolization, and consequent ischaemia (Rose, 1991). According to Rose, few people in Britain reach old age without a potentially dangerous degree of atherosclerosis. Other risk factors, which can influence the severity of atherosclerosis, include: being male, hypertension, hyperlipidaemia, diabetes mellitus, and smoking. Diabetes and smoking are most strongly linked with ischaemia in the legs. Combinations of risk factors, rather than one isolated risk factor, seem to be particularly hazardous.

Atherosclerosis is more common in some sites than in others, commonly affecting the coronary, carotid, and cerebral arteries, with potentially fatal results. In the leg, the most common sites for occlusion are the lower superficial femoral artery (60%), and the aorto-iliac segment (30%), with multiple segment involvement occurring in about 7% of cases (Orr and McAvoy, 1987). The degree of ischaemia and the symptoms experienced depend not only on the site of the occlusion but also on the presence or absence of an effective collateral circulation above and below it. Acute ischaemia due to arterial embolism or trauma (*Table 7*) is potentially the most damaging (as well as life threatening), because the body has not had the time to develop a collateral circulation to compensate. Where an occlusion has developed over a prolonged period of time, it may cause no noticeable effects for the individual.

At rest, an individual may be able to tolerate up to 70% occlusion of an artery in the lower limb without being aware of any ill effects. On exercise, the increased demands for oxygen in the muscles cannot be met, causing *intermittent claudication*. In people with *ischaemic pain at rest*, the blood vessel supplying the area may be 90% occluded. These symptoms of a severely compromised peripheral arterial circulation are very important to look for, and to note, when assessing a patient with a leg ulcer, as will be seen in Section 3.1.1.

A possible relationship between diseases and disorders affecting the arterial system and arterial ulcers is summarised in *Figure 8*. In this schematic representation, tissue ischaemia resulting from a narrowing or distortion of arterioles, or from major vessel stenosis or occlusion, predisposes to necrosis and ulceration following minor trauma. Clinically, the skin surrounding an arterial ulcer is often shiny, and loss of hair, adipose tissue and sweat glands is common, but there is no brown staining in the gaiter area unless there is also chronic venous hypertension.

The significance of an arterial component in leg ulcer aetiology is being increasingly recognised. Both Cornwall *et al.* (1986) and Callam *et al.* (1987a) estimated that about 21% of patients presenting with leg ulcers

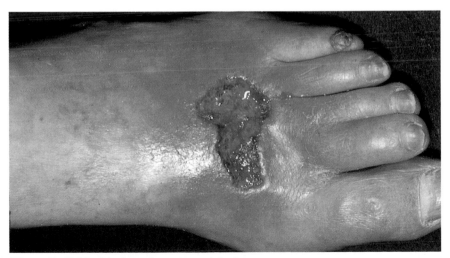

Figure 7. Critical ischaemia: an arterial ulcer.

Table 7. Causes of ischaemia in the leg

- *Atherosclerosis.*
- *Arterial embolism.*
- *Vasospastic diseases*, e.g. Raynaud's.
- *Trauma* e.g. open or closed injuries, such as a leg fracture or dislocation.
- *Cold* e.g. frostbite or immersion injuries.

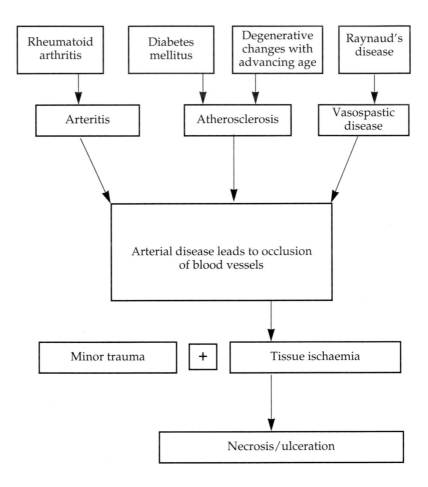

Figure 8. Diseases and disorders associated with arterial ulcers – a tentative model.

have evidence of arterial insufficiency. This has very important implications for treatment (Callam *et al.* 1987b). The accurate, differential diagnosis of venous and arterial leg ulcers is therefore essential (Chapter 3).

2.3   Rheumatoid arthritis and vasculitic ulcers

Leg ulceration is common in patients with rheumatoid arthritis, with up to 10% of patients developing an ulcer at some stage (Pun *et al.,* 1990). The skin overlying the tibia is poorly vascularized in everyone, but is particularly susceptible to trauma and delayed healing in patients with rheumatoid arthritis, especially if they are being treated with high dose corticosteroids. Simply dropping a book off the knees on to the legs, or some other equally minor traumatic incident may lead to an ulcer which takes months to heal.

A deep ulcer in a patient with rheumatoid arthritis is illustrated in *Figure 9*. The underlying vascular problem here is arteritis. Such ulcers tend to appear suddenly, deteriorate rapidly and heal slowly. However, the aetiology of ulcers in patients with rheumatoid arthritis is not always clear (Cawley, 1987). Although often attributed to vasculitis (inflammation of blood vessels), the aetiology may be multifactorial. In a retrospective study over an 8 year period of 33 episodes of leg ulceration in 26 patients with rheumatoid arthritis, Pun *et al.* (1990) found vasculitis to be the cause in only 18.2% of cases. The most common causes were venous insufficiency (45.5%), trauma or pressure (45.5%), and arterial insufficiency (36.4%). In these patients, hospitalisation was prolonged (mean 47.9 days). Even after several attempts, only 42.9% of skin grafts took completely, and the recurrence rate of ulceration was high.

Negus (1991) emphasises the importance of excluding arterial disease in these patients, who may have multiple arterial stenoses and occlusions, which are not suitable for surgery.

Vasculitic ulcers are also associated with some other less common inflammatory connective tissue disorders. They may present as small, often painful multiple ulcers with no indications of chronic venous hypertension. Ulcers such as these may be seen in patients with polyarteritis nodosa, and systemic lupus erythematosus. Diagnosis of the underlying disorder requires a number of special investigations. The erythrocyte sedimentation rate (ESR) is likely to be very high, but this is not specific to vasculitic disorders. Healing of these ulcers is likely to be slow and is very much affected by the course of the underlying disease.

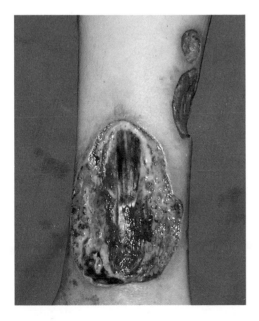

Figure 9. A deep arterial ulcer in a patient with rheumatoid arthritis, with exposed tendon and necrotic tissue visible.
(Ruckley, 1988)

Pyoderma gangrenosum is distinctive, and characterised by acute, necrotising, rapidly expanding ulceration of the skin (*Figure 10*). The ulcer may have an irregular undermined edge and purple margins. There is some doubt as to whether the underlying cause is primarily vasculitic (Pun *et al.*, 1990).

Early referral for further medical assessment is imperative if the nurse suspects vasculitis.

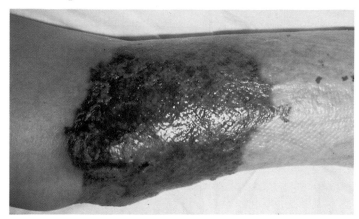

Figure 10. Pyoderma gangrenosum.

2.4   Diabetic ulcers

Ulceration of the lower limb, especially the foot, is a common complication for patients with diabetes mellitus (Robertson *et al.*, 1986). More hospital beds in Britain are occupied by diabetic patients with disorders of their feet than by patients with all the other complications of diabetes combined (Elkeles and Wolfe, 1991). Delayed wound healing and increased vulnerability to infection are likely (Joseph and Axler, 1990), gangrene may develop, and there is a high risk of the need for lower-limb amputation. In the USA it has been estimated that 50% of all non-traumatic amputations occur in diabetic patients, with the elderly at particular risk, and men at significantly higher risk than women of requiring an amputation. Furthermore, the prognosis for the other leg is poor: 42% of patients requiring a second amputation within 1–3 years and 56% within 3–5 years. It has been suggested that 50–75% of these amputations are preventable.

Peripheral sensory neuropathy is probably the most common single cause of foot ulceration in diabetic patients (Young and Boulton, 1991). About one fifth of foot ulcers in diabetics may be due to peripheral vascular disease alone. Very commonly, however, foot ulcers result from a combination of peripheral neuropathy and peripheral vascular disease, and are frequently complicated by infection. Elderly patients living alone are particularly at risk, especially if their vision is impaired and they are unable to inspect their feet daily, as recommended (Section 4.5 and Appendix 5.1). As recurrence is very common, previous foot ulceration should alert the health care professional that the person is at particular risk.

2.4.1 Angiopathy in the diabetic patient

In non-diabetics, occlusion or stenosis is most commonly found in the major arteries of the leg, such as the iliac and femoral arteries. Usually only one leg is involved, only a single segment of the blood vessel is occluded and this may be amenable to bypass surgery (Section 4.5). Peripheral vascular disease in diabetic patients is very common, but the clinical picture is somewhat different.

Occlusion of major arteries may occur (*Figure 11*) but usually it is the more distal, smaller, below-knee vessels which are involved, such as the tibial and peroneal arteries, and more distant branches of these vessels (*Figure 12*). Occlusion is often multisegmental, and both limbs are often affected. Atherosclerotic changes are thought to occur more rapidly in diabetics and to occur at an earlier age (Levin, 1988). Medial calcinosis (calcification of the blood vessels) can be very significant in diabetic patients. The implications of this for non-invasive assessment of the patient's peripheral vascular system are described in Section 3.1.3 and Appendix 3.1.

Risk factors for macrovascular disease in diabetic patients include increasing age, the duration of the diabetes, smoking, hypertension and hypercholesterolaemia. Diabetic patients can suffer adverse changes to small vessels, as well as to the medium and larger arteries.

Disease of the small vessels can give rise to ischaemic damage to the retinae and renal glomeruli, as well as to the digits in the lower limb. The risk

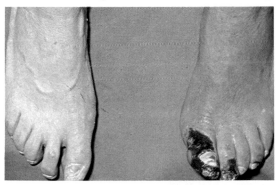

Figure 11. Gangrene of left first and second toes with ischaemia of leg due to occlusion of deep femoral artery.
(Bloom & Ireland, 1992)

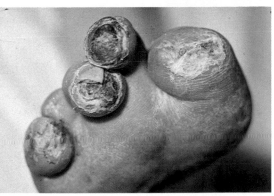

Figure 12. Peripheral ischaemia and dry gangrene associated with occlusion of the arcuate vessels of the dorsalis pedis artery; the necrotic areas gradually demarcate and auto-amputate.
(Bloom & Ireland, 1992)

is greatest in patients whose diabetes is poorly controlled and who experience wild swings between hyperglycaemia and insulin-induced hypoglycaemia.

2.4.2   Neuropathy in the diabetic patient

Three types of peripheral neuropathy occur: sensory, motor and autonomic. For diabetics with *sensory neuropathy,* a reduced or absent pain sensation in the feet can result in unnoticed mechanical, thermal or chemical trauma. Mechanical trauma may be caused by ill-fitting shoes, or stepping on a sharp object. Thermal trauma can arise from too hot a bath, sitting too close to the fire (*Figure 13*), from a hot water bottle, or walking bare foot on a hot surface such as sand. Chemical trauma can occur when diabetics use chemical callus and corn removers.

Motor neuropathy This results in foot deformity due to atrophy of the small muscles of the foot, causing clawing of the toes and prominent metatarsal heads. A changed gait and repeated prolonged pressure can cause a build-up of callus and ulceration on the sole of the foot, especially under the head of the first metatarsal bone (*Figure 14*), over enlarged bunions, and on the bony prominences of the toes (*Figure 15*).

Autonomic neuropathy This results in the absence of sweating, and leads to very dry skin which predisposes patients to develop cracks and fissures, allowing entry of fungi and bacteria.

Unlike most other ulcers of the skin, a neuropathic ulcer, for instance on the plantar surface of the foot, develops initially from deep within the tissues. Fluid collects under the callus, infection follows, leading to abscess formation and ulceration. The opening of the ulcer may at first be small, masking the true extent of deep tissue damage. Infection is a common consequence, often extending down to tendon and bone. If not treated promptly and aggressively (Section 4.5), radical debridement may be required (*Figure 16*).

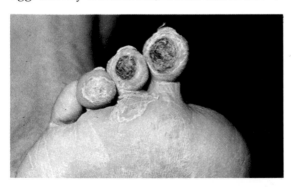

Figure 13. Painless destructive damage to neuropathic toes caused by falling asleep when warming the feet in front of an electric fire. (Bloom & Ireland, 1992)

2.4.3   Other causes of ulceration

Diabetic patients can, of course, also develop ulcers due to chronic venous hypertension (Section 2.1) in the absence of any history, clinical signs, or symptoms of peripheral vascular disease or peripheral neuropathy.

It is crucial to determine the underlying causes of ulceration for each individual. Specialist vascular assessment is particularly important in this group of patients (Section 3.1). More unusual causes of ulceration can also occur in diabetics (Section 2.5).

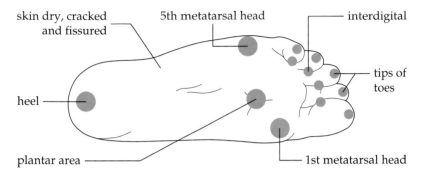

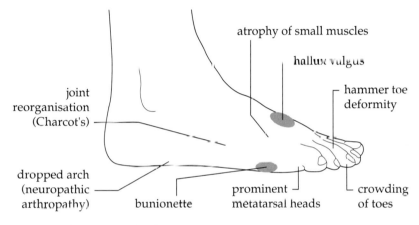

Figure 14. Areas of callus formation and neuropathic ulceration beneath calluses.

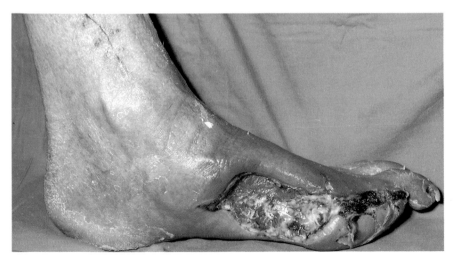

Figure 15. The neuropathic foot.

Figure 16. Radical debridement in a diabetic patient.

There is no such thing as a 'diabetic ulcer', but a diabetic patient with an ulcer which may be due to one or a combination of underlying pathologies.

The diabetic patient's role in preventing ulceration is particularly critical (Section 4.5 and Appendix 5.1), as damage can occur so easily and can have such devastating consequences, whatever the underlying aetiology of the ulcer.

2.5   More unusual causes of leg ulcers

In the majority of patients in the UK presenting with a leg ulcer, the underlying problem is either chronic venous hypertension (Section 2.1), or arterial disease (Section 2.2). People with rheumatoid arthritis may have ulcers primarily due to vasculitis, or to more major arterial occlusion or stenoses (Section 2.3), and delayed healing is common. People with diabetes mellitus can have leg ulcers due primarily to chronic venous hypertension, major artery occlusion or small vessel disease, peripheral neuropathy, or any combination of these problems, as described in Section 2.4. Delayed healing is common in this group too, especially as diabetics are so prone to infection.

Whatever the underlying pathology *appears* to be, it is always important to rule out the more unusual causes of ulceration described below. This is particularly important where the ulcer has resisted all treatments tried over a prolonged period, or if the appearance of the ulcer is unusual.

Many of the tests required to exclude the more uncommon causes of ulceration are beyond the role of the nurse, but as the majority of patients in the UK are assessed and treated by nurses in the community, the nurse has a vital role to play in referring the patient for further assessment if a more unusual cause is suspected. This usually involves referring the patient back to the GP in the first instance, unless the nurse is working in a clinic linked to a vascular or dermatology service, where more specialist assessment may be more readily to hand (Chapter 7).

Malignant ulcers Malignancy is an uncommon cause of ulceration, but the possibility of malignancy should not be overlooked in patients whose ulcers fail to respond to treatment (Ackroyd and Young, 1983). A squamous cell carcinoma can develop in a chronic venous ulcer, and is then known as Marjolin's ulcer. This condition is very rare but should be suspected if the ulcer has an unusual appearance, including, for instance, an overgrowth of tissue in the base or at its margins. It is confirmed by biopsy and histological examination, which should be carried out as a matter of urgency.

Malignant melanoma (*Figure 17*) is more common. It is unlikely to be mistaken for venous ulceration, but it can bear a superficial resemblance to some presentations of Kaposi's sarcoma (*Figures 18a–c*). The malignant form of Kaposi's sarcoma, although currently rare, is becoming more widespread in the western world with the spread of acquired immune deficiency syndrome (AIDS). The lesions are usually small and multiple (*Figure 19*), and can ulcerate.

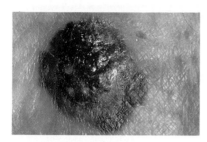

Figure 17. Melanoma.

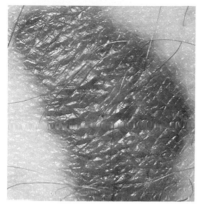

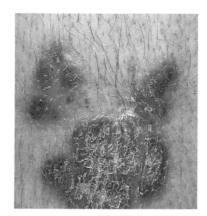

Figures 18a–c. Kaposi's sarcoma lesions from different patients to show variation in colour and appearance. Older lesions are darker and may become scaly.
(Farthing et al., 1988)

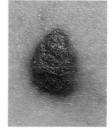

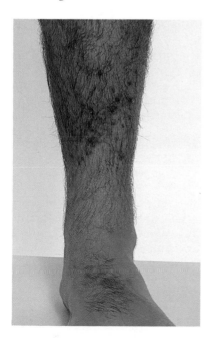

Figure 19. Kaposi's sarcoma presenting on the lower leg, in a patient with AIDS, as in classical Kaposi's sarcoma. About a third of the cases of Kaposi's sarcoma present on the lower leg.
(Farthing et al., 1988)

27

In the tropics, malignant changes are relatively common and appear to develop in ulcers of 12–15 years' duration (Landra, 1988). It is a well known complication of chronic scars following burns, and also of ulcers in the foot of a patient with leprosy.

Blood disorders Leg ulceration can occur in patients with blood disorders such as sickle cell disease and thalassaemia. It often presents as small, multiple, painful ulcers in teenagers and young adults. Polycythaemia is seen in older patients, mostly as atypical ulcers of the foot.

Infection Leg ulcers due primarily to infection, e.g. tuberculosis, syphilis, leprosy and deep fungal infections, are very rare in the UK, but are still seen in people living in, or returning from, the tropics. There, poverty, malnutrition, chronic anaemia, lack of hygienic facilities, and poor medical facilities contribute to delayed healing and a very high incidence of serious complications such as periostitis, osteomyelitis, malignancy and lymphoedema. Tropical ulcers which are due to mixed infections are a very common problem in young adults and military personnel operating overseas, and for people in refugee camps; in fact, anywhere where poverty and a warm and humid climate coexist (Landra, 1988).

Although, to date, lower leg ulceration is not definitively associated with HIV disease the HIV-positive patient is more prone to skin disorders such as seborrhoeic dermatitis, xeroderma and psoriasis which can affect the legs. Skin lesions due to a number of causes can break down in the AIDS patient. Kaposi's sarcoma can also ulcerate. Because of their immunocompromised status and the presence of concurrent debilitating conditions, often including a poor nutritional status, delayed healing, especially from infections, is almost inevitable in these patients, and in some cases wounds may never heal (Cohen and Prystowski, 1992). There is an increased risk of secondary infection, often by unusual organisms or organisms that are not normally pathogenic.

Walzman *et al.*'s (1986) case report of leg ulceration due to syphilitic osteomyelitis of the tibia of an 81 year old lady with peripheral vascular disease emphasises the importance of thorough assessment for all cases of intractable ulceration. This may necessitate a period of hospitalisation while vascular and other investigations are performed.

Metabolic disorders Ulceration in patients with diabetes mellitus has already been considered (Section 2.4). Ulceration of the lower limb is not uncommon in patients with pyoderma gangrenosum.

Lymphoedema Lymphatics are the drains which remove large molecules of fat and protein from the tissues, as well as cells and excess fluid (Ryan, 1987). In venous disorders, the superficial lymphatic vessels can be excessively dilated and damaged, and the accumulation of waste products causes low grade inflammation and fibrosis, and predisposition to cellulitis. Elephantiasis is due to a combination of venous insufficiency and lymphatic fibrosis (*Figure 20*). It involves gross thickening of the dermis (*Figure 21*). An early sign is stiffness of the tissues of the dorsum of the toes, which can be felt when attempting to pinch the skin.

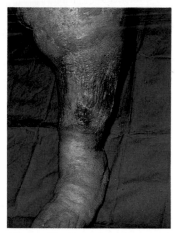

Figure 20. Lymphoedema and obesity.

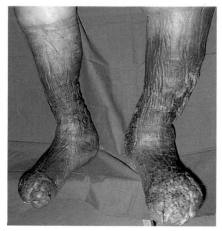

Figure 21. Chronic venous hypertension and damage to the lymphatic vessels have led to gross thickening of the dermis.

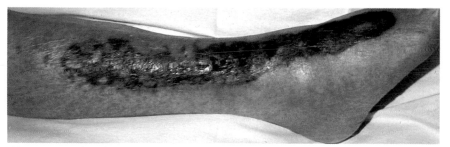

Figure 22. A bandage-induced ulcer which led to amputation. (Ruckley, 1988)

Trauma Where there is an underlying vascular problem, minor trauma can lead to an intractable ulcer. In this case, the minor traumatic event, which could be a minor knock to the leg, or an insect bite, is merely a final trigger leading to tissue breakdown. In people who do not have an underlying peripheral vascular problem, more major trauma can lead to a period of ulceration. The skin overlying the tibia is poorly vascularized even in healthy people, and a sizeable traumatic pretibial laceration can take some time to heal, especially if there is tissue loss or care is not taken to remove contaminating debris or haematoma, prior to closure of the wound with skin tapes. The risk of infection following a dog bite to the leg is high, and if the bite was inflicted by a human, is even higher.

The management of minor traumatic wounds is described by Morison (1992) and Grossman (1992) and is beyond the scope of this book.

Iatrogenic ulcers Inadequate patient assessment, especially the failure to identify a significant degree of arterial impairment, can lead to inappropriate management of the limb, and at worst precipitate its amputation (*Figure 22*). This will be discussed in more depth in Section 4.1, where the hazards of applying compression are considered. Even when sustained compression of the lower limb is not contraindicated, over-tight bandaging can lead to pressure necrosis over bony prominences. Pressure damage can also be induced by an inexpertly applied lower limb cast.

Self-inflicted injury Much has been written about the 'social ulcer'. An attempt to present a balanced view of self-inflicted injury as a possible cause of delayed ulcer healing, and other factors to consider, is given in Section 4.7.5. The proportion of patients who interfere with an ulcer with the express purpose of gaining attention and continued care is unknown. The 'natural' recurrence rate for leg ulceration is sadly very high (Section 1.1), but the extent to which this is influenced by a patient's deliberate infliction of further trauma to a recently healed ulcer is unknown.

Further reading

The following texts have been selected because they give a particularly authoritative review of the subject and are useful for background reading. Most are also excellent sources of further illustrations, including both common and more unusual clinical presentations of leg ulcers.

Anatomy and physiology of the peripheral circulation (arterial and venous)

Seeley, R.R., Stephens, T.D. & Tate, P. (1992) *Anatomy and Physiology* (2nd edn) Mosby–Year Book, St. Louis, pp. 645–697.

Anatomy of the veins of the lower limb

Negus, D. (1991) The anatomy of the veins of the lower limb. In: Negus, D. *Leg ulcers: a practical approach to management*. Butterworth–Heinemann, Oxford, pp. 14–26.

Mechanisms of venous return from the lower limb

Negus, D. (1991) Venous return from the lower limb muscle pumps: normal and disordered function. In: Negus, D. *Leg ulcers: a practical approach to management*. Butterworth–Heinemann, Oxford, pp. 27–36.

Diabetic foot ulcers

Bloom, A. & Ireland, J. (1992) *A Colour Atlas of Diabetes* (2nd edn) Wolfe Publishing, London.

Boulton, A.J.M. (1988) The diabetic foot. *Med Clin North Am* **72(6)**, 1513–1530.

Levin, M.E. (1988) The diabetic foot: pathophysiology, evaluation and treatment. In: Levin, M.E. & O'Neal, L.W. (eds) *The diabetic foot* (4th edn) CV Mosby, St. Louis, pp. 1–50.

Vasculitis and ulceration in rheumatic diseases

Cawley, M.I. (1987) Vasculitis and ulceration in rheumatic diseases of the foot. *Bailliere's Clin Rheumatol* **1(2)**, 315–333.

Conn, D.L. (ed) (1990) Vasculitic syndromes. *Rheum Dis Clin North Am* **16(2)** (whole issue).

HIV and AIDS

Farthing, C.F., Brown, S.E. & Staughton, R.C.D. (1988) *A Colour Atlas of AIDS and HIV disease* (2nd edn) Wolfe Medical Publications, London.
Neal, S. & Penneys, S. (1990) *Skin manifestations of AIDS* Martin Dunitz

The tropical ulcer

Landra, A.D. (1988) The tropical ulcer. *Surgery* **59**, 1402–1403.

References

Ackroyd, J.S. & Young, A.E. (1983) Leg ulcers that do not heal. *BMJ* **286**, 207–208.
Bloom, A. & Ireland, J. (1992) *A Colour Atlas of Diabetes* (2nd edn) Wolfe Publishing, London.
Browse, N.L. & Burnand, K.G. (1982) The cause of venous ulceration. *Lancet* **ii**, 243–245.
Burnand, K.G., Whimster, I., Naidoo, A. & Browse, N.L. (1982) Pericapillary fibrin in the ulcer-bearing skin of the leg: the cause of lipodermatosclerosis and venous ulceration. *BMJ* **285**, 1071–1072.
Callam, M.J., Harper, D.R., Dale, J.J. & Ruckley, C.V. (1987a) Arterial disease in chronic leg ulceration: an underestimated hazard? Lothian and Forth Valley Leg Ulcer Study. *BMJ* **294**, 929–931.
Callam, M.J., Ruckley, C.V., Dale, J.J. & Harper, D.R. (1987b) Hazards of compression treatment of the leg: an estimate from Scottish surgeons. *BMJ* **295**, 1382.
Cawley, M.I. (1987) Vasculitis and ulceration in rheumatic diseases of the foot. *Bailliere's Clin Rheumatol* **1(2)**, 315–333.
Cohen, J.I. & Prystowski, J.H. (1992) Treatment of ulcerated HIV-associated Kaposi's sarcoma with combination chemotherapy. *Wounds* **4**, 208–214.
Coleridge Smith, P.D., Thomas, P., Scurr, J.M. & Dormandy, J.A. (1988) Causes of venous ulceration: a new hypothesis. *BMJ* **296**, 1726–1727.
Cornwall, J., Dore, C.J. & Lewis, J.D. (1986) Leg ulcers: epidemiology and aetiology. *Br J Surg* **73**, 693–696.
Dalziel, K.L. & Bickers, D.R. (1992) Skin aging. In: Brocklehurst, J.C., Tallis, R.C. & Fillit, H.M. (eds) *Textbook of Geriatric Medicine and Gerontology* (4th edn) Churchill Livingstone, Edinburgh, pp. 898–921.
Elkeles, R.S. & Wolfe, J.H.N. (1991) The diabetic foot. *BMJ* **303**, 1053–1055.
Farthing, C.F., Brown, S.E. & Staughton, R.C.D. (1988) *A Colour Atlas of AIDS and HIV disease* (2nd edn) Wolfe Medical Publications, London.
Gardner, A.M.N. & Fox, R.H. (1986) The return of blood to the heart against the force of gravity. In: Negus, D. & Jantet, G. (eds) *Phlebology '85*. Libbey, London, pp. 65–67.
Grossman, J.A.(ed) (1992) *Atlas of minor injuries and repairs* Gower Medical Publishing, London.
Herrick, S.E., Sloan, P., McGurk, M., Freak, L., McCollum, C.N. & Ferguson, M.W.J. (1992) Sequential changes in histological pattern and extracellular

matrix deposition during the healing of chronic venous ulcers. *Am J Pathol* **141(5)**, 1085–1095.

Joseph, W.S. & Axler, D.A. (1990) Microbiology and antimicrobial therapy of diabetic foot infections. *Clin Podiatr Med Surg* **7(3)**, 467–481.

Landra, A.D. (1988) The tropical ulcer. *Surgery* **59**, 1402–1403.

Levin, M.E. (1988) The diabetic foot: pathophysiology, evaluation and treatment. In: Levin, M.E. & O'Neal, L.W. (eds) *The diabetic foot* (4th edn) CV Mosby, St. Louis, pp. 1–50.

Morison, M.J. (1992) Traumatic wounds. In: Morison, M.J. *A colour guide to the nursing management of wounds* Wolfe Publishing, London, pp. 186–203.

Negus, D. (1991) *Leg Ulcers: A Practical Approach to Management* Butterworth–Heinemann, Oxford.

Orr, M.M. & McAvoy, B.R. (1987) The ischaemic leg. In: Fry, J. & Berry, H.E. (eds) *Surgical Problems in Clinical Practice* Edward Arnold, London, pp. 123–135.

Pun, Y.L.W., Barraclough, D.R.E. & Muirden, K.D. (1990) Leg ulcers in rheumatoid arthritis. *Med J Aust* **153(10)**, 585–587.

Robertson, J.C., Daunt, S.O'N. & Nur, M. (1986) Tissue viability – wound healing and the diabetic. *Practical Diabetes* **3**, 14–19.

Rose, G. (1991) Epidemiology of atherosclerosis. *BMJ* **303**, 1537–1539.

Ruckley, C.V. (1988) *A colour atlas of surgical management of venous disease* Wolfe Medical Publications, London.

Ryan, T.J. (1987) *The management of leg ulcers* (2nd edn) Oxford University Press, Oxford.

Seeley, R.R., Stephens, T.D. & Tate, P. (1992) *Anatomy and Physiology* (2nd edn) Mosby–Year Book, St. Louis, pp. 645–697.

Thomas, P.R.S., Nash, G.B. & Dormandy, J.A. (1988) White cell accumulation in dependent legs of patients with venous hypertension: a possible mechanism for trophic changes in the skin. *BMJ* **296**, 1693–1695.

Walzman, M., Wade, A.A.H., Drake, S.M. & Thomas, A.M.C. (1986) Rest pain and leg ulceration due to syphilitic osteomyelitis of the tibia. *BMJ* **293**, 804–805.

Young, M.J. & Boulton, A.J.M. (1991) Guidelines for identifying the at-risk foot. *Practical Diabetes* **8(3)**, 103–105.

3. Patient assessment

3.0   Introduction

When a patient presents for the first time with a leg ulcer, a general patient assessment is required to determine:

- The *immediate cause* of the ulcer.
- Any underlying *pathology* in the lower limb.
- Any *local problems at the wound site* which may delay healing.
- Other more general *medical conditions* which may delay healing.
- The patient's *social circumstances* and the optimum setting for care.

3.1   Assessing the immediate cause of the ulcer and any underlying pathology

When taking a patient's history the *immediate cause* of the ulcer should be determined. For most patients, the immediate cause of tissue breakdown is a minor traumatic event. For a person with diabetes mellitus who has peripheral neuropathy, the ulcer may be due to ill-fitting footwear (Section 2.4). It is important to determine the immediate cause of the ulcer to facilitate the development of a plan, with the patient, to prevent recurrence (Section 4.1.8). It is of paramount importance to *go on* to determine any *underlying pathology* in the lower limb which could make the patient prone to delayed healing and to recurrent ulceration if uncorrected.

Assessment of the patient's clinical signs and symptoms, past medical history, and some simple investigations, normally give sufficient information for the nurse to decide whether the patient is presenting with an ulcer due to:

- Chronic venous hypertension (about 70% of cases).
- Arterial disease (about 10% of cases).
- A combination of chronic venous hypertension and arterial disease (10–20% of cases).

The differential diagnosis of the more unusual causes of ulceration, such as haemoglobinopathies and metabolic disorders (Section 2.5), is beyond the scope of this book, and beyond the nurse's responsibility.

If there is any doubt about the underlying aetiology of an ulcer, the nurse is strongly advised to refer the patient to a doctor as soon as possible, to arrange for a further assessment.

Specialist assessment is particularly important for patients with diabetes mellitus, where the consequences of mismanagement can be so disastrous, and for patients with suspected arterial disease, where a thorough vascular assessment is required to determine the nature and extent of the problem, and whether or not the person is a suitable candidate for vascular surgery.

Criteria for referral of leg ulcer patients to the Vascular Surgical Service, developed at Charing Cross Hospital in London, are given in *Table 8.*

Table 8. Criteria for referral of leg ulcer patients to the Charing Cross Vascular Surgical Service

- Patients found to have a *resting pressure index of 0.5 or below* should be referred **immediately** to the Vascular Surgical Service. Patients should be seen within one week of referral. *(No compression to be applied.)*
- Patients with a *resting pressure index between 0.5 and 0.8* should also be referred for vascular opinion.
- Patients with an index of 0.6–0.7 may receive reduced compression. See Criteria for Reduced Compression.
- *Young, mobile patients* should be referred for a full venous assessment with a view to simple vein surgery.
- Patients with *recurrent ulceration* should be considered for referral for full venous assessment, and possible surgery to avoid further recurrence.
- *All ulcers failing to make satisfactory progress* should be referred to the Vascular Surgical Service.
- Patients presenting with *ulcers where a more unusual cause is suspected* should be referred for full investigation.

3.1.1 Clinical signs and symptoms

The clinical signs and symptoms of venous and arterial disorders in the lower limb were described in Sections 2.1.2 and 2.2, and are summarised in *Tables 9* and *10.* An explanation of the underlying pathophysiology which gives rise to these signs and symptoms is given in Chapter 2, which discusses the mechanisms leading to ulceration.

Interpretation of the *symptoms* of vascular disease requires considerable clinical experience. Problems causing pain with walking, such as arthritis, must be differentiated from intermittent claudication. The non-ischaemic causes of pain with walking however, usually take longer to disappear than claudication pain. It is also important to note that, while intermittent claudication most commonly occurs as pain in the calf, high level vascular obstruction can cause pain in the buttocks and thighs and may be accompanied by impotence.

Table 9. Venous problems: clinical signs and symptoms

1. *Prominent superficial leg veins or symptoms of varicose veins, such as:*

    - *Aching or heaviness* in legs, generalised or localised.
    - Mild ankle *swelling*.
    - Itching over *varices*.
    - Symptoms due to thrombophlebitis, localised *pain, tenderness* and *redness*. (Gentle exercise such as walking round the room or repeated heel raising helps to show distension of the veins.)

2. *Ankle flare.* Distension of the tiny veins on the medial aspect of the foot below the malleolus

3. *Pathological changes to the skin and tissues surrounding the ulcer, including:*

    - *Pigmentation* 'Staining' of the skin around the ulcer.
    - *Lipodermatosclerosis* Hardening of dermis and underlying subcutaneous fat, which may feel 'woody'.
    - *Stasis eczema*
    - *Atrophe blanche* Ivory white skin stippled with red 'dots' of dilated capillary loops.

4. *Site of ulcer* Frequently near the medial malleolus, sometimes near the lateral malleolus, but can be anywhere on the leg.

Table 10. Arterial problems: clinical signs and symptoms

1. Whole leg/foot
   Symptoms:

    - *Intermittent claudication:* cramp-like pain in the muscles of the leg, brought on by walking a certain distance (depending partly on speed, gradient and patient's weight). The patient gains relief by standing still to rest the ischaemic calf muscles.
    - *Ischaemic rest pain:* intractable constant ache felt in the foot, typically in the toes or heels. Usually relieved by dependency: hanging the leg over the bed or sleeping upright in a chair.

   Signs (many are suggestive but not specific to ischaemia):

    - *Coldness of the foot.*
    - *Loss of hair.*
    - *Atrophic, shiny skin.*
    - *Muscle wasting in calf or thigh.*
    - *Trophic changes in nails.*
    - *Poor tissue perfusion, e.g. colour takes more than 3 seconds to return after blanching of toenail bed by applying direct pressure*
    - *Colour changes: foot/toes dusky pink when dependent, turning pale when raised above the heart.*
    - *Gangrene of toes.*
    - *Loss of pedal pulses.*

2. Site of ulcer

    - Usually on the foot or lateral aspect of the leg but may occur anywhere on the limb, including near the medial malleolus, which is the most common site for venous ulcers.

Rest pain usually indicates at least two significant arterial stenoses or occlusions in series. It decreases with dependency of the lower limb and is made worse by heat, elevation and exercise. In the course of peripheral vascular disease, nocturnal, ischaemic pain usually precedes rest pain. It occurs at night during sleep when peripheral perfusion is reduced. The person gains relief by dangling the feet over the edge of the bed. In diabetic patients, severe pain in the legs at night can be due to diabetic neuropathy or vascular insufficiency, or both.

The signs and symptoms of *acute* arterial occlusion are given in *Table 11. Irreversible damage* to skeletal muscle and peripheral nerves occurs within 4–6 hours of severe ischaemia, in the absence of an adequate collateral circulation.

Patients known to have severe peripheral vascular disease must be warned to seek immediate medical help should they develop sudden extreme pain in the leg.

For the diabetic patient, peripheral neuropathy is the most significant cause of ulceration. The neuropathy may be sensory, motor or autonomic. The signs and symptoms of diabetic neuropathy are summarised in *Table 12*. An explanation of the underlying pathology

Table 11. Clinical signs and symptoms of acute arterial occlusion in the lower limb

- *Pain* of sudden onset and severe intensity.
- *Pallor*.
- *Paraesthesia* (numbness).
- *Pulselessness* (absence of pulses below the occlusion).
- *Paralysis* (sudden weakness in the limb).
- *Polar* (a cold extremity).

Table 12. Clinical signs and symptoms of neuropathy in the diabetic foot and leg

1. Foot deformity e.g. hammer toes, Charcot's foot with collapse of the metatarsal joints giving a 'club foot' appearance.

2. Excessive callus formation over bony pressure points, e.g. under the metatarsal heads and the plantar surface of the foot.

3. Altered sensation (paraesthesia).

   - *Hyperaesthesia* Excessive sensitivity of the feet which may be so great that the individual cannot bear the slightest touch. The pain may be constant and is often more severe at night.

   or

   - *Hypoaesthesia* Diminished sensitivity to pain, vibration, temperature or position. The foot may feel 'dead' or the individual may report unusual sensations when walking for example, likening it to walking on cushions.

4. Reduced or absent sweating, often accompanied by dry skin with cracks and fissures.

which gives rise to these signs and symptoms is given in Section 2.4, where a number of common clinical presentations are also illustrated. Diabetic neuropathy is frequently bilateral and tends to be symmetrical. Patients are inclined to under-report symptoms of reduced sensation (hypoaesthesia) unless specifically questioned, yet knowledge of such symptoms is crucially important for planning appropriate care and attempting to prevent recurrence of ulceration.

It is important to note that there are causes of peripheral neuropathy other than diabetes mellitus. These include alcoholism, collagen disorders, pernicious anaemia, malignancy affecting the spinal cord, and uraemia.

The importance of *specialist* vascular assessment for patients thought to have a significant degree of peripheral arterial disease, and for patients with diabetes mellitus, cannot be overemphasised.

3.1.2 Past medical history

Table 13 summarises the factors in a patient's past medical history which may throw some light on the underlying vascular problems which led to the development of the ulcer.

Chronic venous hypertension is suggested by a history of varicose veins with valve incompetence, which may have been precipitated by any one or more of a number of thrombogenic events, e.g. leg fracture, immobility post-surgery, or during pregnancy (see *Figure 5* and Section 2.1).

Callam *et al.* (1987) found that a history of stroke, transient ischaemic attacks, angina or myocardial infarction increased the probability of *arterial* impairment in the lower limb, and a history of intermittent

Table 13. Past medical history: indicators of possible venous or arterial problems

1. Indicators of possible venous problems
    *   Previous thrombogenic events
        Has the patient ever suffered from one or more of the following:

        *   Deep vein thrombosis.
        *   Thrombophlebitis.
        *   Leg or foot fracture in the affected limb?.

    *   Varicose veins

        *   Does the patient have prominent superficial leg veins, with signs of valve incompetence?
        *   Has the patient ever had any varicose vein surgery or sclerotherapy in the affected leg?

2. Indicators of possible arterial problems
    *   Generalised arterial disease

        Are there any indicators of arterial disease such as:
        *   Previous myocardial infarction.
        *   Angina.
        *   Transient ischaemic attacks.
        *   Intermittent claudication.
        *   Cerebrovascular accident.

claudication was almost invariably associated with poor peripheral perfusion.

3.1.3   Some simple vascular assessment methods

3.1.3.1 Palpation of foot pulses In the past, *the presence of palpable foot pulses* has been taken as a sign of unimpaired arterial circulation in the lower limb, and the *absence* of pulses as indicative of arterial impairment. This is not an entirely fail-safe test for several reasons.

In a recent study, where community nurses palpated pulses in 533 ulcerated limbs, no pulses were detectable in 25% of cases where another simple vascular assessment indicated that it would have been safe to apply compression. 37% of patients with detectable pulses were demonstrated to have significant peripheral arterial disease. In this study, lack of pedal pulses had a positive predictive value for significant arterial disease in only 35% of cases! (Moffatt *et al.*, 1993)

This is not just a matter of academic interest. If a patient has a venous ulcer but no palpable foot pulses, withholding compression therapy in the mistaken belief that the patient has a significantly impaired peripheral arterial circulation would inevitably delay healing, as the underlying problem of chronic venous hypertension would not be corrected.

It is important to note that *the dorsalis pedis pulse is congenitally absent in up to 12% of individuals* (Barnhorst and Barner, 1968). If the dorsalis pedis pulse is not felt, it is important to palpate the posterior tibial pulse (*Figure 23*). Oedema is a common problem in patients with ulcers, and this can make pulses hard to feel.

There are a number of other clinical situations where the *presence* of pedal pulses can give a false impression of a good peripheral arterial circulation, as the following three examples illustrate:

- Clinical examination of patients complaining of intermittent claudication involving the calf muscle may reveal both femoral and pedal pulses, but no popliteal pulse. In this case, the pedal pulses are present at rest if there is a good collateral circulation, but they disappear when the patient takes a brisk walk if the peripheral circulation is considerably compromised. The treadmill test (Appendix 3.1) is a useful test in these circumstances, to confirm the presence of significant arterial impairment and the need for further specialist investigations.
- In diabetic patients, pedal pulses may be palpable, but this does not rule out the possibility of a severely compromised blood supply more distally, to the toes, which if left untreated could lead to irreversible tissue damage and the need for amputation. Palpable pedal pulses are usually present in patients with small vessel disease, unless there is coexisting and severe atherosclerosis.
- Finally, even though the posterior tibial vessel is occluded and the pulse here is absent, and there is significant local ischaemia in the region of the medial malleolus, the dorsalis pedis pulse may still be present. This can occur, for example, when the person has suffered local trauma to the lower limb.

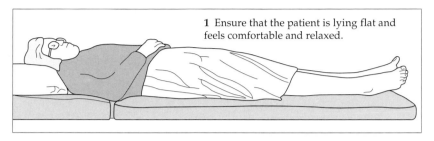

1 Ensure that the patient is lying flat and feels comfortable and relaxed.

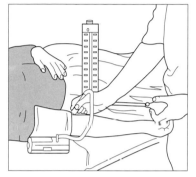

2 Secure sphygmomanometer cuff around arm.

Apply ultrasound gel over brachial pulse.

Hold Doppler probe gently over brachial pulse until a good signal is obtained.

Inflate cuff until Doppler signal disappears then gradually lower pressure until the signal returns. This is the Brachial Systolic Pressure Record. (Diastolic pressure is not recordable with Doppler)

3 Examine the foot for posterior tibial and dorsalis pedis pulse using fingers and/or Doppler probe.

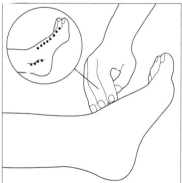

4 Secure sphygmomanometer cuff just above ankle.

Locate posterior tibial or dorsalis pedis pulse using Doppler probe and gel.

Inflate cuff until signal disappears, then gradually reduce pressure until the signal returns.
This is the Ankle Systolic Pressure.
(Spuriously high readings may be obtained in elderly or diabetic patients as the cuff may not fully compress the calcified vessels.)

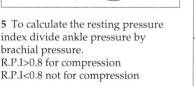

5 To calculate the resting pressure index divide ankle pressure by brachial pressure.
R.P.I>0.8 for compression
R.P.I<0.8 not for compression

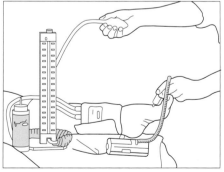

Figure 23. The procedure for recording the resting pressure index (RPI), sometimes referred to as the ankle brachial pressure index (ABPI). (Based on Moffatt & Stubbings, 1990.)

The above examples illustrate the danger of basing a diagnosis on a single subjective test. The non-invasive vascular assessment tests described below can confer objective significance to the findings detected on clinical examination, the patient's reports of symptoms, and any indicators of venous or arterial problems in the patient's past medical history.

3.1.3.2 **The resting pressure index (RPI) test** A simple vascular assessment technique, which can be readily carried out by nurses following a period of supervised practice, is the *resting pressure index* (RPI) test. This is sometimes referred to as the *ankle brachial pressure index* (ABPI) test and it is a very useful starting point in patient assessment.

It involves determining the ratio of the ankle to the brachial systolic pressure, with the aid of a simple hand-held, battery-operated Doppler ultrasound probe in place of a stethoscope.

$$\text{Resting pressure index (RPI)} = \frac{\text{ankle systolic pressure}}{\text{brachial systolic pressure}}$$

The procedure for recording the resting pressure index is illustrated in *Figure 23*.

To overcome the effects of previous exercise on blood pressure, the patient should lie as flat as possible for at least ten minutes. During this time, the patient's history can be taken and the brachial systolic pressure measured in the usual way, in the right arm. Patients with dyspnoea may not be able to lie completely flat. This should be recorded. Any open ulcerated area can be covered with a simple dressing.

To assess the ankle systolic pressure, the cuff is sited just above the malleolar area and the pressure measured using either the posterior tibial or dorsalis pedis pulse (*Figure 23*). The angle at which the Doppler probe should be held, as recommended by the manufacturers, ranges from 45–60°. In practice, the angle may need to be adjusted if the vessel does not run parallel with the skin. A good seal between the probe and the skin is critical. This is the reason for using the acoustic coupling gel. A beam of sound waves, emitted by a crystal in the probe, travels to the underlying blood vessel where it is reflected from red blood cells in proportion to the flow velocity of the cells. The returning signal is picked up by a second crystal in the probe. Different probes can be used for different purposes. The higher the frequency emitted by the crystal (measured in MHz), the less the depth of penetration. A 1–5 MHz frequency probe is usually used for monitoring deep blood vessel flow, while a 6–10 MHz probe is ideal for determining blood flow in more superficial vessels of the limbs and digits. In a noisy clinic, and for patients with significant peripheral arterial disease, headphones can be very useful.

The RPI allows for individual variations in blood pressure, and should normally be greater than 1.0. Patients with a ratio of 0.9–0.95

probably have some degree of arterial disease. If the RPI is less than 0.8 there is significant impairment in the arterial blood supply, which means that compression bandaging is contraindicated, and further vascular assessment is required. A ratio of 0.5–0.75 is often associated with intermittent claudication, and < 0.5 with ischaemic rest pain. A rapid referral to a doctor is advisable if the index is below 0.75.

A resting pressure index above 1.2 may be pathological, for instance in a patient with medial calcinosis. In diabetic patients a falsely high RPI may be obtained for this reason, as the blood vessels are very difficult to compress.

If there is any doubt about the significance of the RPI the doctor should be consulted for further advice.

3.1.4 Other simple investigations

Some simple investigations which can yield valuable results are summarised in *Table 14*.

A wide range of clinical and objective tests for the assessment of the diabetic foot (which may be carried out in a specialist clinic), including tests for pain, vibration and proprioception is described by Boulton (1988) and Levin (1988).

Table 14. Other simple investigations

- *BM stix* to detect the possibility of undiagnosed diabetes, which is often associated with peripheral arterial problems.
- *Blood tests* to test for rheumatoid and antinuclear factors which may indicate potential arteritis or auto-immune disorders; full blood count and estimation of haemoglobin levels.
- *Patch testing for allergens,* e.g. lanolin and parabens, which are present in many commonly used wound care products.
- *Tissue biopsy* if malignant changes are suspected.
- *Wound swabs* to identify the nature and antibiotic sensitivity of any organisms causing clinical signs of infection.

3.1.5 Further vascular assessment methods

The physician may decide to request a specialist vascular assessment, especially if localised occlusion of a blood vessel, which might be amenable to surgery is suspected. Criteria for referral to a vascular surgical service are given in *Table 8*.

The role of the Non-invasive Vascular Investigation Unit has changed dramatically over the past twenty years. Originally, only a recording of the resting pressure index (RPI) was routinely carried out. The range of investigations has been revolutionised by the use of *colour-coded, duplex ultrasound scanners* which are able to provide real-time moving images, not only revealing the location and extent of vessel lumen stenosis, but also enabling blood-flow velocity measurements. These tests are at present only available in specialist centres.

41

Invasive radiological procedures such as arteriography and venography, which were the mainstay of vascular assessment, but which carry a relatively high risk of complications, are now generally reserved for patients undergoing surgery.

A typical pathway for a patient presenting for assessment at the Charing Cross clinic is given in *Figure 24*. Details of some of the more specialist tests are given in Appendix 3.1. A comprehensive and well illustrated summary of more specialist diagnostic methods is given in Negus (1991). Williams *et al.* (1993) describe how relatively simple Doppler ultrasound techniques can be used to confirm a clinical diagnosis, or to detect the severity of arterial insufficiency. Picton *et al.* (1993) describe how both the deep and the superficial venous systems can be assessed using hand held Doppler probes.

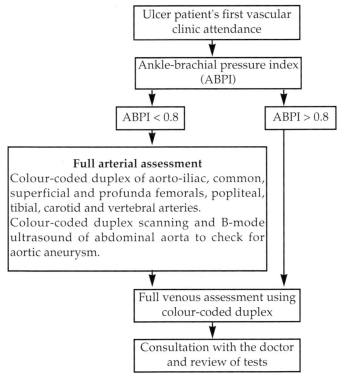

Figure 24. The Charing Cross protocol for patient assessment within the Vascular Surgical Service.

3.1.6 Mixed aetiology ulcers

Between 10% and 20% of leg ulcers do not fall neatly into either the venous or arterial categories. A patient's leg may show all the classic signs of chronic venous hypertension, but there may also be underlying arterial problems. The checklist in *Table 15* can be used to help determine whether the ulcer is likely to be of venous, arterial or mixed aetiology.

Table 15 Differential diagnosis of venous and arterial leg ulcers: some points to consider when assessing patients (tick boxes that apply to the patient; the pattern of ticks should give some indication of the underlying aetiology of the ulcer)

Indicators of venous problems

1. *Past medical history*
   - Has the patient ever suffered from any of the following: deep vein thrombosis, thrombophlebitis or leg/foot fracture in the affected limb? ☐
   - Has the patient ever had any varicose vein surgery or sclerotherapy in the affected limb? ☐

2. *Clinical signs and symptoms in the leg*
   - Prominent superficial leg veins. ☐ ☐
   - Brown pigmentation of the skin around and just above the ankle. ☐
   - Distension of the tiny veins in the medial aspect of the foot. ☐
   - Lipodermatosclerosis (hard 'woody' induration of the lower leg). ☐ ☐
   - Stasis eczema.
   - Atrophe blanche (skin thin, white and stippled with red dots).

3. *Simple vascular assessment/tests*
   - Pedal pulses present. ☐ ☐
   - Resting pressure index (RPI) > 0.9.

Indicators of arterial problems

1. *Past medical history*
   - Are there any indicators of generalised arterial disease, e.g. myocardial infarction, angina, transient ischaemic attacks, intermittent claudication, cerebrovascular accident? ☐

2. *Clinical signs and symptoms in the leg*
   - Intermittent claudication. ☐ ☐ ☐ ☐
   - Ischaemic rest pain.
   - Pain relief when the leg is lowered below heart level.
   - Foot dusky pink when dependent, turning pale when elevated above the heart. ☐ ☐
   - Poor tissue perfusion, e.g. colour takes more than 3 s to return after blanching of toenail bed by applying direct pressure. ☐
   - Loss of hair, atrophic shiny skin. ☐

3. *Simple vascular assessment/tests*
   - Pedal pulses absent or very faint indeed. ☐ ☐
   - Resting pressure index (RPI) < 0.9.

A small percentage of leg ulcers are not due to vascular problems. If the wound has an unusual appearance, is in an unusual site or is refractory to healing, or if the patient has recently arrived in the UK from abroad, or is a teenager, a more unusual cause should be suspected (see Section 2.5).

If the nurse is unsure of the underlying cause of any ulcer, she should refer the patient to a doctor for further assessment without delay.

3.2 Local wound assessment

After assessing the underlying cause of the ulcer, assessment of the wound itself should be undertaken, as this may determine the method of wound cleansing, and the most appropriate primary wound contact dressing.

It is helpful to *trace* the ulcer every 2–4 weeks using an acetate sheet or transparent glove, and a fine permanent marker pen. The tracing can be annotated with information such as the nature of the wound bed and wound margins, the date, and the patient's name (*Figure 25*). Tracing ulcers is one useful guide to evaluating the effectiveness of treatment, but the inherent inaccuracies in this simple method should not be forgotten (Johnson, 1993). Wounds are three-dimensional. The surface area of an ulcer may change little, although healing is progressing well, with the wound granulating from beneath and reducing in depth. The surface area may also increase as the wound is debrided. Plassmann and Jones (1992) describe a colour-coded, structured light technique for the three dimensional measurement of leg ulcers. Such levels of sophistication are, however, rarely available in the clinical setting.

Offensive odour, the general condition of the surrounding skin, the nature and severity of pain at the wound site or elsewhere, the possibility

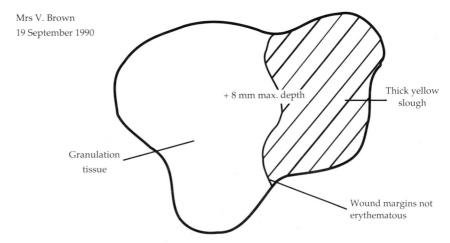

Figure 25. Leg ulcer tracing.

of infection, and whether or not a wound swab has been sent for culture and antibiotic sensitivity testing should be noted, as should any previous allergies to wound care products. The reasons for pain at the wound site should be very carefully assessed (*Table 16*). So many of these causes are easily correctable, and correction can significantly improve the quality of the patient's life.

Charting the healing of leg ulcers (*Figure 26*) is a very helpful aid to evaluating the effectiveness of local wound treatment. If a leg ulcer shows no signs of healing it may be because:

- The local problems at the wound site have not been dealt with appropriately.
- The underlying cause of the ulcer has not been identified and corrected.
- Some other patient factor is delaying healing.

Table 16. Possible causes of pain at the wound site and at dressing changes

---

Pain is a common accompaniment of leg ulcers of many aetiologies, including venous hypertension. If the patient complains of pain at the wound site or experiences pain at dressing changes, the nurse should consider the following:

1. Pain at the wound site

- *Is the wound infected?* Look for other local and systemic signs and symptoms of clinical infection, especially if the onset of pain is sudden.
- *Is any overlying conforming or compression bandage too tightly applied?* Has the bandage slipped? Are there tight bands of constriction overlying the wound or over any nearby bony prominences?
- *Is there underlying ischaemia?* For example, in a patient with severe peripheral vascular disease even small open wounds can be very painful and there may be rest pain in the limb. In patients with atrophe blanche, small ulcers can also be extremely painful, possibly due to ischaemia in the microvascular bed.

2. Pain at dressing changes

- *Is the dressing adhering, causing tissue trauma on removal?* Even low-adherent dressings can adhere to the wound if they are left in place for too long, especially if exudate strikes through the dressing and then dries out. Fresh bleeding on dressing removal is an obvious sign of trauma.
- *Is the most painless method of dressing removal being employed?* Removal of adhesive dressings or the tapes used to hold a dressing in place can be very painful if removal is against the lie of any hair present. Removing dressings and tapes in line with the hairs is virtually painless. If a dressing has adhered to the wound bed it should be gently soaked off, not ripped off 'quickly'.
- *Is a cleansing solution being used that could be causing an irritant tissue response,* such as a hypochlorite?
- *Is the nurse lacking in empathy?* Is the nurse underestimating the significance of the wound to the individual?

Open Wound Assessment Chart

Type of wound (ε.γ. venous or arterial leg ulcer)..

Location...

How long has wound been open?..

General patient factors which may delay healing (ε.γ. malnourished, diabetic, chronic infection)...

....

Allergies to wound care products...

Previous treatments tried (comment on success/problems)...

a. Debridement..

b. Primary dressings..

....

....

TRACE THE WOUND EVERY TWO WEEKS, ANNOTATING TRACING WITH MAXIMUM DIMENSIONS (length, breadth), NATURE OF WOUND BED, ORIENTATION OF WOUND
All other parameters should be assessed at **every** dressing change and changes documented.

Wound factors/Date								
1. NATURE OF WOUND BED a. healthy granulation b. epithelialisation c. sloughy d. hard black necrotic e. others (specify)								
2. EXUDATE a. colour b. amount: heavy/moderate/ minimal/none								
3. ODOUR Offensive/some/none								
4. PAIN (SITE) Specify								
5. PAIN (FREQUENCY) Continuous/intermittent/ only at dressing changes/none								
6. PAIN (SEVERITY) Patient's score (0–10)								
7. WOUND MARGIN a. colour b. oedematous?								
8. ERYTHEMA OF SURROUNDING SKIN a. present b. max. distance from wound (mm)								
9. GENERAL CONDITION OF SURROUNDING SKIN (wet or dry eczema)								
10. INFECTION a. suspected b. wound swab sent c. confirmed (specify organism)								
WOUND ASSESSED BY:								

Figure 26. Open wound assessment chart.

3.3 Other factors that may affect healing

When taking the patient's history and carrying out an assessment of the patient's current general physical condition, it is worth noting any other factors that could contribute to delayed wound healing such as:

- Evidence of, or suspected, *malnutrition.*
- *Poor mobility,* of whatever cause, which may adversely affect the calf muscle pump and venous return.
- An *occupation,* or activities, that involve prolonged standing, especially in warm conditions.
- *Decreased resistance to infection,* whatever the cause.
- Poor *social* circumstances.

The range of local and systemic factors known to affect healing are summarised in *Figure 27.* While the effects of increasing age *per se* cannot be overcome, good wound healing is possible even in very elderly patients (Section 1.4), and advanced age should not be used as an excuse for merely maintaining the status quo.

In addition to a thorough physical assessment, assessment of the patient's psychosocial problems is also very important. The check list given in *Table 17* is a useful tool for summarising the positive and negative psychosocial factors relevant to an individual. The patient's occupation and social circumstances should be considered when deciding on the practical arrangements for managing the ulcer.

Table 17. Assessment of positive and negative psychosocial factors which can affect recovery from any illness. (Tick boxes which apply to patient and add any particularly relevant information below.)

Positive Factors		Negative Factors	
Good knowledge of illness/condition	☐	Unwilling or unable to know about illness/condition	☐
Active participation in treatment	☐	Lack of belief in, and unwillingness to participate in, treatment	☐
Good relationships with staff	☐	Poor relationships with staff	☐
Flexible coping methods	☐	Passive dependence, persistent denial or highly emotional disposition	☐
Good supportive social relationships	☐	Poor family relationships, living alone	☐
Positive orientation to treatment and rehabilitation from members of the health care team (hospital and/or community)	☐	Negative attitudes of staff to treatment and healing	☐
		Additional recent life stress, e.g. bereavement, separation, loss of employment	☐

Other information:

_____

_____

_____

_____

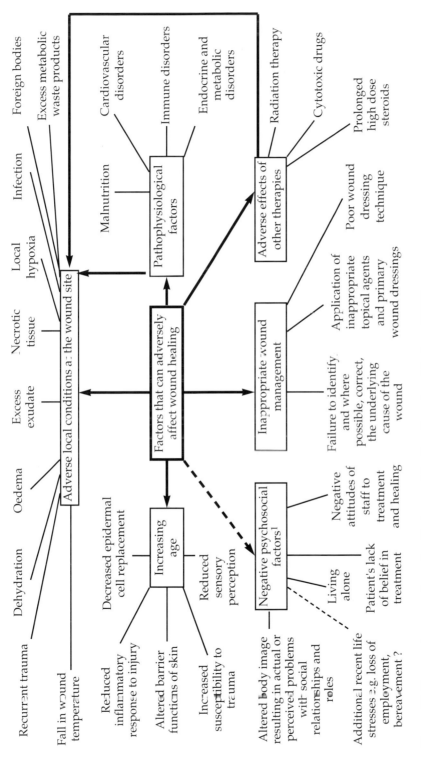

Figure 27. *Factors that can adversely affect wound healing (based on Morison, 1992).*
Note: [1] *The direct link between delayed healing and negative psychosocial factors has yet to be unequivocally demonstrated.*

Appendix 3.1 More specialist vascular assessment

This appendix outlines some of the more common procedures carried out within a vascular laboratory. Facilities will vary greatly throughout the country. Nurses should be familiar in outline with the techniques described, in order to be able to explain to patients what may be involved if they are referred for a specialist assessment. A brief indication of the precautions and hazards is given.

A. Arterial assessment

Patients presenting with an ulcer thought to be of arterial aetiology require a full vascular investigation. In addition to the resting pressure index test (Section 3.1.3.2), the following tests may be undertaken:

1. Non-invasive arterial assessment procedures

Treadmill exercise test Patients presenting with a history of claudication but with a resting pressure index (RPI) above 0.8 are asked to perform an exercise test on a treadmill. Patients are exercised for one minute, at 4.00 Km/hr at an angle of 10°. They then revert to the supine position (in which the RPI was initially measured), and the ankle–brachial pressure index (ABPI) is recorded approximately 40 seconds after the cessation of the exercise. If the ABPI falls below 0.8, significant arterial disease is indicated, requiring a more extensive arterial assessment. This test is unsuitable for patients with poor mobility, severe unstable angina, or cardiac disease.

Segmental pressures Segmental pressures are used to help to assess the location of significant arterial occlusions and stenoses in the lower limbs. Recordings of the blood pressure are taken using a Doppler probe placed over a distal vessel, and cuffs placed at different levels on the limb:

- High thigh .
- Low thigh.
- High calf.
- Ankle.

A pressure drop of 30 mmHg, or more, between segments indicates severe disease or occlusion of the artery between these points. Segmental pressure measurements are particularly useful in patients with calcified arteries. Examples of typical segmental pressure readings, and their clinical significance, are illustrated in the Table opposite.

Position of pressure cuff	Segmental pressures in 4 patients (figures given for one side of the body only)			
	1	2	3	4
Arm	180	145	140	160
Leg A. High thigh	190	200	190	174[2]
B. Low thigh	180	180	180	90[2]
C. High calf	180	160	166	70
D. Ankle	180	230	142[1]	50
E. Toe [3]	NA	NA	60[1,3]	NA
Ankle/arm index (RPI)	$\frac{180}{180}$=1.00	$\frac{230}{145}$=1.59	$\frac{142}{140}$=1.01	$\frac{50}{160}$=0.31
Underlying problem	Normal No problems detected	Medial calcification leading to abnormally high RPI in a diabetic patient Vessels patent. Oedema	Small vessel disease in big toe (Note: normal RPI)	Superficial femoral artery obstruction

Notes: NA = not available

[1, 2] The difference in these readings is particularly significant. Any gradient greater than 30 mmHg between two successive cuffs usually indicates high-grade stenosis or occlusion (Hurley *et al.* 1988).

[3] Toe signals are difficult to detect, requiring the use of a pencil probe. The results obtained can be very useful clinically but this measurement is only undertaken in a few specialist centres.

Listening to and observing wave forms is important and can give a clue to normality (see Williams *et al.*, 1993). Interpretation of these measurements is more difficult when there is multilevel involvement.

Colour-coded duplex scanning of the peripheral arteries With the help of a colour-coded duplex scanner it is possible to visualise blood vessels from the aorta to the ankle, and to detect the site and degree of stenosis or occlusion in them. It involves using an ultrasound machine that is able to portray the blood vessels and surrounding tissues in blacks, greys, and white (the B-mode picture). It is also able to overlay the moving blood in colour on the same picture. Different directions and speed of blood flow can be shown using different colours.

B-mode scanning of the abdominal aorta The normal aortic diameter is 1.5–2.0 cm and can be measured with simple B-mode ultrasound. If the diameter is greater than 3.0 cm, the patient has an abdominal aortic aneurysm. This may rupture or embolise and occlude the distal vessels.

Carotid and vertebral colour-coded duplex scanning The extracranial cerebral vessels are scanned to check degrees of stenosis, as these may indicate the risk of stroke.

2. Invasive arterial assessment procedures

Angiography Patients undergoing arterial surgery normally have arteriography to confirm the extent of the disease. This provides useful anatomical information about the arterial system from the upper aorta to the pedal vessels, and complements non-invasive investigations. It is usually reserved as a pre-operative investigation. Radio-opaque dye is injected into the femoral artery.

Arteriography is not without risk. The risks include an anaphylactic reaction to the dye, renal shutdown, thrombus formation at the injection site, haematoma and peripheral emboli.

B. *Venous assessment*

1. Non-invasive venous assessment procedures All patients with venous ulcers should have a resting pressure index recorded to identify any arterial component (Section 3.1.3.2). This risk rises considerably with age, with 50 per cent of patients at risk of arterial disease when aged over 75 years. Various invasive and non-invasive tests to assess venous function are described below.

Colour-coded duplex ultrasound This is used to assess both deep and superficial venous systems. The veins are visualised as the calf is gently squeezed, forcing blood upwards towards the heart and thus allowing assessment of the function of each vein. The normal flow in a well-functioning vein is easily distinguished from the abnormal reflux of blood caused by non-functioning valves in incompetent deep and perforating veins. The presence of deep vein thrombosis can also be detected. This method is now considered to be the gold standard.

Portable Doppler ultrasound This can be used to assess venous reflux, as well as for identifying arterial disease. Sites of incompetence can be detected at various sites from the groin to the calf. The Doppler probe is held over the vein and the calf gently squeezed, producing upward flow. On relaxation, no flow should be heard when valves are functioning normally. Sites may be missed, particularly if there is a variation in anatomy. Some of the methods used are described in more detail by Picton *et al.* (1993).

Air plethysmography This is used to assess both venous reflux, and deep vein thrombosis and obstruction. Air plethysmography detects volume changes in the calf, using an air-filled cuff placed on the calf. This, however, is a very time consuming procedure.

Photoplethysmography This is a relatively simple, non-invasive procedure which uses infra-red light to measure the time taken for the superficial veins to refill after exercise. In severe venous disease, this time is shortened as blood rapidly refluxes through the damaged valves.

Photoplethysmography is often used as a screening procedure to detect venous disease, and to differentiate superficial from deep vein reflux.

Foot vein pressure (AVP: ambulatory venous pressure) This is used to assess calf pump function, and involves cannulation of a foot vein and attachment to a pressure chart recorder. The patient performs ten tiptoe exercises or a standard exercise test, to empty the calf of venous blood. Normally, venous pressures fall after exercise. The veins are filled by the arteries and capillaries, and return to pre-exercise levels in not less than 20 seconds. The pressure recorded at the end of the exercise is the ambulatory venous pressure. When venous disease is present and reflux occurs, the venous pressure drops only slightly, indicating that exercise is unable to empty the veins and reduce the venous pressure effectively. Tourniquets may be used to occlude superficial veins at different levels, in order to assess the relative contribution of deep and superficial function independently. This is a difficult, lengthy procedure. It is not suitable for patients with reduced mobility.

2.   Invasive venous assessment procedures

Venography This was once the most commonly used method to assess venous disease, but it is much less frequently used today due to the development of very powerful non-invasive methods. Contrast medium is injected into the femoral vein to outline the venous system. Venography can be used to detect acute thromboses, chronic occlusion of the deep veins and incompetent perforating veins. While giving anatomic information it sheds no light on peripheral haemodynamics directly. It is an expensive and lengthy procedure.

As with arteriography, venography is potentially a hazardous procedure with the risk of an anaphylactic reaction to the contrast medium. It involves exposure to radiation and it can be painful for the patient.

An excellent summary of more specialist diagnostic methods is given by Negus (1991).

References

Barnhorst, D.A. & Barner, H.B. (1968) Prevalence of congenitally absent pedal pulses. *N Engl J Med* **278**, 264–265.

Boulton, A.J.M. (1988) The diabetic foot. *Med Clin North Am* **72(6)**, 1513–1530.

Callam, M.J., Harper, D.R., Dale, J.J. & Ruckley, C.V. (1987) Chronic ulcer of the leg: clinical history. *BMJ* **294**, 1389–1391.

Hurley, J.J., Hershey, F.B., Auer, A.I. & Binnington, H.B. (1988) Non-invasive evaluation of peripheral arterial status: the physiologic approach. In: Levin, M.E. & O'Neal, L.W. (eds) *The diabetic foot.* (4th edn) CV Mosby, St. Louis, p. 119–130.

Johnson, A. (1993) Wound assessment. *Wound Management* **4(1)**, 27–30.

Levin, M.E. (1988) The diabetic foot: pathophysiology, evaluation and treatment. In: Levin, M.E. & O'Neal, L.W. (eds) *The diabetic foot* (4th edn) CV Mosby, St. Louis, pp. 1–50.

Moffatt, C.J., Oldroyd, M.I., Greenhalgh, R.M. & Franks, P.J. (1993) The use of ankle pulses in detection of arterial insufficiency in patients with leg ulceration. Abstract, 3rd European Conference on advances in wound management, Harrogate 1993.

Moffatt, C.J. & Stubbings, N. (1990) The Charing Cross approach to venous ulcers. *Nursing Standard (supplement)* **5(12)**, 6–9.

Morison, M.J. (1992) Wound care (RCN Nursing Update Supplement). *Nurs Stand* **6(37)**, 9–14.

Negus, D. (1991) Diagnosis: methods of investigation. In: Negus, D. *Leg ulcers: a practical approach to management* Butterworth–Heinemann, Oxford, pp. 61–87.

Picton, A.J., Williams, I.M. & McCollum, C.N. (1993) The use of Doppler ultrasound 2: venous disease. *Wound Management* **4(1)**, 13–15.

Plassmann, P. & Jones, B.F. (1992) Measuring leg ulcers by colour-coded structured light. *Journal of Wound Care* **1(3)** 35–38.

Williams, I.M., Picton, A.J. & McCollum, C.N. (1993) The use of Doppler ultrasound 1: arterial disease. *Wound Management* **4(1)**, 9–12.

4. Treatment options

4.0 Priorities in leg ulcer management

Thorough, systematic and accurate assessment of the patient, the identification of the underlying cause of the ulcer (Section 3.1) and any local problems at the wound site (Section 3.2), are prerequisites to planning appropriate care and to preventing avoidable delays in healing. The main management priorities are:

- To *correct* the underlying cause of the ulcer. This normally means improving the patient's venous and/or arterial circulation in the affected limb.
- To *create* the optimum local environment at the wound site.
- To *improve* all the wider factors that might delay healing, especially poor mobility, malnutrition and psychosocial issues.
- To *prevent* avoidable complications such as wound infection, medicament dermatitis, or tissue damage due to over-tight bandaging.
- To *maintain* healed tissue.

The principles behind the management of venous, arterial and mixed aetiology ulcers are now described, with the emphasis on correcting the underlying cause of the ulcer. The principles of the management of ulcers associated with rheumatoid arthritis are outlined in Section 4.4, and the management of diabetic foot ulcers is described in Section 4.5. Creating the optimum local environment for healing is discussed in Section 4.6, and ways of correcting or alleviating the effects of general patient factors that can delay healing are discussed in Section 4.7. The assessment and management of any patient with a leg ulcer requires a team approach, in which the *patient* is a key player. Patient education and ways of encouraging compliance with treatment are discussed in Chapter 5.

4.1 Management of venous ulcers

4.1.1 Aims of management

The main cause of venous ulceration is chronic venous hypertension, with very high pressures being exerted on the superficial venous system, usually due to incompetent valves in the deep or perforating veins (Section 2.1). The primary aims of venous ulcer management are therefore:

- To *reduce* blood pressure in the superficial venous system.
- To *aid* venous return of blood to the heart, by increasing the velocity of flow in the deep veins.
- To *reduce* oedema by reducing the pressure difference between the capillaries and the tissues.

The best way of achieving these aims is to apply *graduated compression* from the base of the toes to the knee. Methods of achieving graduated compression include the application, to the lower limb, of:

- *Bandages,* e.g. Blue Line, Tensopress, Setopress, Veinopress, Elastocrepe.
- *Shaped elasticated tubular bandages,* e.g. Tubigrip.
- *Compression stockings,* e.g. Venosan, Sigvaris, Jobst, Medi (UK).

Each method has advantages and disadvantages, as indicated in *Table 18* and described below.

4.1.2 Characteristics of compression bandages

It is very important to know the performance characteristics of a wide range of compression bandages, if a bandaging regime is to be selected which meets the patient's needs. The advantages and disadvantages of a number of widely available compression and support bandages are summarised in *Table 19* and reviewed by Moffatt (1992).

There are basically two types of compression bandage:

- Those containing an *elastomer,* such as rubber or Lycra, as in Elset, Tensopress and Blue Line. These are capable of exerting medium to very high compression on the limb.
- Those *without elastomer,* which rely on crimped cotton, wool, or rayon threads for their extensibility, such as Elastocrepe and all types of crepe bandage. Lower sub-bandage pressures are obtainable with these bandages.

The elasticity of the bandage determines:

- How much tension is necessary to achieve the required pressure.
- How well the bandage will maintain this pressure.
- Its conformability to the awkward contours of foot, ankle and leg.

Sub-bandage pressure Some of the factors affecting the pressure that can be achieved under a bandage are given in the following equation:

$$P \text{ is proportional to } \frac{N \times T}{C \times W}$$

where
- P is the pressure exerted by the bandage;
- N is the number of layers of bandage;
- T is the bandage tension;
- C is the circumference of the limb;
- W is the bandage width.

The practical implications of the relationships in this equation will now be described.

Number of layers of bandage It can be predicted from the above equation that the more layers applied to the leg, the higher the sub-bandage pressure obtained, and the more likely it is that the pressure will be sustained for prolonged periods. Having said this, good, well sustained compression can be obtained with some single layer bandaging regimens. For example,

Table 18. Methods of achieving graduated compression

Method	Advantages	Disadvantages
1. Bandages	• Can be left *in situ* for up to a week in the absence of excess exudate, except for highest compression bandages e.g. Blue Line. • By varying the tension under which the bandage is applied, the pressure can be varied to suit individual needs and tolerances. • A range of bandages is available in the community. • Relatively low initial cost.	• Excessively high pressures can be obtained with the heavy compression bandages, especially on thin legs and over bony prominences. • Not cosmetically acceptable to many, leading to low compliance. • Uncomfortable in hot weather. • May require patient to purchase a larger size of shoe to accommodate bandage • Some prone to slip, leading to tight bands.
2. Shaped, elasticated, tubular bandages	• Two layers toe to knee useful in patients who cannot tolerate an elastic compression bandage. • Can help to reduce bandage slippage when used over a medium-light compression bandage.	• Not concurrently available in the community. • Only slightly increases the pressures obtained when applied over a bandage; little sustained compression achieved when applied alone.
3. Elastic compression stockings	• Pressure profiles of stockings are tested and known. • A range of compression profiles is available to meet individual needs. • Much safer than inappropriately applied heavy compression bandages. • Cosmetically acceptable • Useful in preventing recurrence of ulceration.	• Require proper fitting for length, ankle and calf size. • Initial cost is high, but compares well with the cost of elastic compression bandages over 6 months. • Difficult for patients with restricted movement to apply themselves. • Compliance rate variable; high compression stockings often poorly tolerated by the elderly but well liked by younger patients who are more mobile.

Table 19. Advantages and disadvantages of a number of commonly used compression and support bandages

Type of bandage	Examples (Manufacturers)	Advantages	Disadvantages
1. *Non-adhesive extensible bandages* Very high compression	Blue Line (Seton); Elastoweb (Smith + Nephew)	a. High pressures obtainable, suitable for counteracting venous stasis in the lower limb for active patients with venous ulcers (RPI $\geq$ 0.9 and preferably $\geq$ 1.0). b. Can be washed and reused.	a. High risk of tissue necrosis over bony prominences if inexpertly applied, especially to a thin leg. b. Must be taken off at night and reapplied in the morning, therefore suitable only for patients who can apply the bandage themselves. c. Cosmetically unacceptable to some patients.
Medium–high compression	Tensopress (Smith + Nephew); Veinopress (Steriseal); Setopress (Seton)	a. Good compression, well sustained, suitable for patients with venous ulcers (RPI $\geq$ 0.9). b. Less risk of pressure necrosis than with very high compression bandages. c. Can be worn continuously for up to one week. d. Comfortable and conformable. e. Can be washed and reused.	High pressures can be obtained over thin legs, therefore potentially hazardous if inexpertly applied; padding may be required.
Light compression/light support	Elastocrepe (Smith + Nephew); Litepress (Smith + Nephew)	a. Elastocrepe useful over paste bandages; increasing pressure achieved and pressure maintained over time (RPI $\geq$ 0.8).	a. Low pressures obtained; used alone it gives only light support. b. A single wash reduces pressures obtained with

Light support only Crepe (many manufacturers)	Performance improved when covered with shaped elasticated tubular bandage which helps to prevent bandage slippage. b. Used as layer 3 in a 4-layer technique (Table 21) and for control of oedema. Useful only for: a. Holding dressings in place. b. As one of several layers in a multilayer bandage in treatment of venous ulcers. c. For light support of minor strains and sprains.	Elastocrepe by about 20%. c. Bandage slippage can occur.
2. *Cohesive extensible bandages* Cohesive bandages Co-plus (Smith + Nephew); Coban (3M); Secure forte (Johnson & Johnson); Lestreflex (Seton)	a. Adhere to themselves, preventing slippage, therefore useful over non-adhesive bandages such as Elastocrepe, and over paste bandages. b. Compression well sustained. Suitable for patients with an RPI ≥ 0.85–0.9.	a. Pressures obtained are too low to be effective in management of venous ulcers. b. 40–60% of bandage tension (and hence pressure) lost in first 20 min after application. . Can be hazardous in inexperienced hands as can cause tight bands round ankle and damage to tendons if wrongly applied.
3. *Hydrocolloid adhesive compression bandages* Hydrocolloid compression bandage Granuflex adhesive compression bandage (Convatec)	a. Good compress on, well maintained (RPI > 0.8). b. Comfortable and conformable. c. Hydrocolloid can greatly improve condit on of skin surrounding ulcers. d. Little slippage.	Not recommended for very fragile skin or where there is extensive wet eczema.

very good compression has been reported for the hydrocolloid adhesive compression bandage (*Table 19*), which is sustainable for 6–7 days (Sockalingham *et al.*, 1990).

A number of multilayer bandage regimens are described in the next section (Section 4.1.3). Some multilayer regimens, such as the four-layer bandage system designed at Charing Cross Hospital (*Table 20*) have been demonstrated to achieve excellent healing rates (Section 1.4).

Bandage tension The bandage tension is proportional to:

- The *elasticity* of the bandage.
- How much the bandage is *stretched* when it is applied.
- How many times the bandage has been *washed*.
- How *long* the bandage has been in place.

It is very important to adhere to the manufacturer's recommendations concerning the tension to be achieved when applying the bandage. If the manufacturer's recommendations are exceeded, dangerously high pressures may be achieved, which could lead to tissue necrosis over bony prominences.

Limb circumference The circumference of the limb also affects sub-bandage pressure. As the pressure exerted by the bandage is *inversely* proportional to the circumference of the leg, the thinner the leg the higher the pressures obtainable:

Dangerously high pressures can be achieved with very high compression bandages in frail, elderly patients with thin legs, especially over bony prominences such as the malleolus and the tibia, and over the tendinous prominences around the ankle (*Figure 22*).

Conversely, it is difficult to achieve high compression on a wide diameter leg, especially one with thick adipose tissue. It is therefore very important to consider limb circumference when selecting a bandage. Two examples of recommended bandage combinations for different ankle circumferences are given in *Tables 20* and *21*. More details of these regimens and how to apply compression bandages are given in the sections which follow.

When seeking to aid venous return, *graduated* compression is required, with the highest pressure at the ankle (30–40 mmHg), gradually decreasing to about 50% of this pressure just below the knee. Since most legs are considerably narrower at the ankle than at the knee, graduated compression is *automatically* achieved if the bandage is applied at the *same tension* all the way up the leg. If, however, the gradient between the ankle and the below-knee circumference is too steep, as in the classic 'inverted champagne bottle' shape of leg, it may be helpful to apply extra padding at the ankle to facilitate the application of safe, therapeutic, graduated compression.

Bandage width The pressure exerted by a bandage is inversely proportional to its width. Higher pressures are therefore obtained with narrower bandages, and lower pressures with wider ones. A 10 cm bandage is

Table 20. The four-layer bandage system designed at Charing Cross Hospital: bandage combinations, according to ankle circumference, for patients with venous ulcers (Moffatt, 1992, p.48). The ankle circumference should be measured on first assessment and the measurement repeated one week later, when the oedema has reduced.

Ankle circumference	Bandages
Less than 18 cm	2 or more Velband 1 crepe 1 Elset 1 Coban
18–25 cm	1 Velband 1 crepe 1 Elset 1 Coban
25–30 cm	1 Velband 1 Plastex 23 1 Coban
Greater than 30 cm	1 Velband 1 Elset 1 Plastex 23 1 Coban

Table 21. Another four-layer bandage regimen for venous ulcer management. The ankle circumference should be measured on first assessment and the measurement repeated one week later, when the oedema has reduced.

Ankle circumference	Bandages
Less than 18 cm	2 or more Soffban Natural 1 Propax Crepe 1 Litepress 1 Co-plus
18–25 cm	1 Soffban Natural 1 Propax Crepe 1 Litepress 1 Co-plus
25–30 cm	1 Soffban Natural 1 Tensopress 1 Co-plus
Greater than 30 cm	1 Soffban Natural 1 Litepress 1 Tensopress 1 Co-plus

appropriate in most cases. Care should be taken to overlap bandages evenly, with each turn of the bandage overlapping its predecessor by half the bandage width to give an even pressure gradient.

The advantages and disadvantages of a range of compression bandages are given in *Table 19*. As new products for community use are regularly being added to the Drug Tariff, it is advisable to check which bandages are currently available.

4.1.3 Multilayer bandaging regimens

In the previous section, it was seen that one way of increasing sub-bandage pressure is to apply more than one layer of bandage.

The first four-layer bandaging regimen to be extensively tested was developed at Charing Cross Hospital in London. The regimen is summarised in *Table 20*. All the bandages are applied from the base of the toes to just below the knee. The first layer of orthopaedic wool is applied in a spiral. This layer absorbs exudate and redistributes pressure around the ankle, protecting bony prominences and filling in the troughs behind the malleoli where little pressure would otherwise be exerted. The second layer, also applied in a spiral, is a cotton crepe bandage which adds absorbency and smoothes the orthopaedic wool layer, thus preserving the elastic energy of the layers which follow. For most patients, who have an ankle circumference of 25 cm or less, the third layer is Elset. This is a highly elastic, conformable compression bandage which is applied as a figure of eight with a 50% overlap. The final layer is Coban. This is a lightweight, elastic, cohesive bandage which is durable and maintains the bandage layers in place. It is applied in a spiral.

For patients with ankles measuring 25–30 cm the crepe and Elset bandages are substituted by Plastex 23. This is a strong elastic bandage which is applied in a spiral.

A small proportion of patients with obesity or lymphoedema have ankles measuring in excess of 30 cm. For these patients, Elset, Plastex 23 and Coban are applied over the first layer of orthopaedic wool.

Limb circumference may change during the first few weeks of treatment, particularly if the patient had been suffering from gross oedema. With any regimen determined on the basis of ankle circumference, the ankle should be remeasured weekly to ensure that the patient receives the correct regimen.

Another four-layer regimen which is undergoing extensive clinical trials is summarised in *Table 21*.

Other three-layer regimens which can give excellent healing results include an elastic regimen consisting of wool padding (Soffban natural)/elastic lycra bandage (Tensopress)/graduated tubular bandage (Tensoshape), and a non-elastic regimen comprising wool padding (Soffban natural)/cotton bandage (Elastocrepe)/cohesive bandage (Co-plus). A recent study found that the elastic compression regimen just described was more effective than the non-elastic regimen, and was better tolerated by patients, who experienced less pain.

For some patients with chronic skin disorders, a paste bandage may be indicated (*Table 22*). Several layers are applied over the ulcerated area, and the paste bandage is folded back over itself over the bony prominences to prevent excessive pressure here, and to allow the leg room to expand should it become oedematous, as may happen in hot weather, or if the patient stands in one place for too long (*Figure 28*).

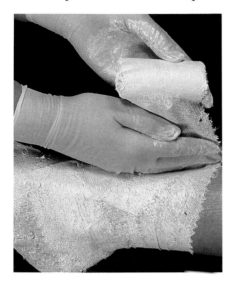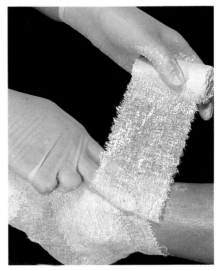

Figure 28a, b. Application of a paste bandage. After each turn around the limb, fold and apply in the opposite direction, until the skin is covered to just below the knee. (Stone et al., 1989)

Table 22. Paste bandages

Principal constituents	Proprietary name (Manufacturer)	Indications
Zinc paste	Viscopaste PB7 (Smith + Nephew); Zincaband (Seton)	General purpose treatment for leg ulcers, venous stasis, eczema and chronic dermatitis. Soothing. Sensitivity reactions relatively infrequent.
Zinc paste and calamine	Calaband (Seton)	Emollient properties, soothing and hydrating for dry, scaly lesions surrounding leg ulcers. Can be applied over ulcer itself.
Zinc paste and ichthamol	Ichthopaste (Smith + Nephew); Icthaband (Seton)	Wet ulcers surrounded by sensitive skin. Soothing and mildly keratolytic. Ichthamol has a milder action than coal tar and is useful in less acute forms of eczema.
Zinc paste and coal tar	Coltapaste (Smith + Nephew); Tarband (Seton)	Dry, itchy eczema where the skin surface has not broken down. Coal tar relieves itching and has keratolytic properties.

A double layer of tube gauze can be applied over the paste bandage before continuing with the multilayer principle, e.g. wool padding/ elastic lycra bandage/graduated tubular bandage. Paste bandages are soothing, and can rehydrate the skin surrounding the ulcer. Unfortunately, some contain ointment bases and preservatives that lead to sensitivity reactions in certain patients (Section 4.6.2.6.).

4.1.4 Criteria for using reduced compression

Before any treatment is begun, a full assessment of the patient should be carried out (Chapter 3) to eliminate the possibility that the patient also has an arterial problem, with poor peripheral perfusion in the affected leg.

Criteria for using reduced compression, based on the protocols developed for use by the Riverside Community Leg Ulcer Clinics are given in *Table 23*.

A number of bandaging regimens can be used in these situations. Examples include:

- Wool padding/crepe/Elset.
- Wool padding/Elastocrepe/shaped elasticated tubular bandage.

Reduced compression should be used with great care, and modified according to the patient's symptoms and resting pressure index.

If in doubt about the advisability of applying compression to the limb, always seek a medical opinion.

Referral criteria for specialist vascular assessment are given in *Table 8*.

Table 23. Criteria for use of reduced compression in patients suffering with leg ulcers (Riverside Community Leg Ulcer Clinics)

- Full compression using the four-layer bandage is suitable only for patients with a resting pressure index of 0.8 or above.
- Reduced compression can be considered in selected patients with a pressure index of 0.6–0.7. This should comprise Velband/crepe/Elset only. These patients should be closely monitored and referred for a vascular opinion.
- Patients with diabetes may have falsely elevated pressure indices. Diabetics with reduced pressure indices should **not** receive compression. These patients should also be referred for specialist opinion.
- No patient with a pressure index of 0.5 or less should receive compression bandaging.
- All patients with reduced pressure indices should be 're-Dopplered' at 3 month intervals or if symptoms change.

4.1.5 Applying the bandage

Applying a compression bandage safely and effectively requires considerable skill and much practice. It is important to practise bandaging technique on colleagues before applying bandages to patients. If possible, it is helpful during training to borrow a sub-bandage pressure monitoring device to record the pressures obtained at several points on the leg. One method of gaining a 'feel' for the pressures to be obtained is to inflate a sphygmomanometer cuff round the ankle to 40 mmHg, and then move it up to the upper calf and inflate it to 20–25 mmHg. The cuff should feel pleasantly firm and supportive but not too tight.

Before applying the bandage, it is important that both the patient and the nurse are positioned comfortably. Bending over a patient's leg can cause considerable back strain. Ideally, the patient should be positioned on a couch or padded trolley with the foot at right angles to the leg and at a height which is comfortable for the nurse to work at. In the patient's home, a high foot stool and pillows may achieve the best position. The use of a chiropodist's stool by the nurse should also be considered. All the materials required should be arranged so that they are within easy reach.

When applying any compression to the lower leg, it is important to include the base of the toes and to apply the bandage to just below the knee. Graduated compression can be obtained by applying the bandage at the same tension all the way up the leg, after suitably padding bony prominences. Some bandages include a simple visual guide to facilitate application of the bandage at the correct tension. *Figure* 29 shows how to apply a bandage in a spiral, beginning with the base of the toes, incorporating the heel, and filling in under the foot before spiralling up the leg. *Figure 30* illustrates how to apply a figure of eight bandage. Ulcers occurring in the hollow behind the malleolus may receive inadequate compression. Local pressure can be increased here by placing a foam or gauze pad between the first and second bandage layers, over the ulcer site.

Whichever bandaging regimen is used, care should be taken to overlap bandages evenly to prevent tight bands over bony prominences. Where bandages overlap, the pressure is higher than where there is a single layer of bandage. It is therefore important that each turn of the bandage overlaps its predecessor by half the bandage width to give an even pressure gradient. When the bandage is removed, no deep grooves or indentations should be seen. Bandage damage can precipitate amputation, especially in ischaemic limbs where compression is contraindicated.

4.1.6 *Compression stockings*

Compression stockings are used to control oedema, in the management of varicose veins, and in the prevention and treatment of ulcers due to chronic venous hypertension. They have a number of advantages over bandages (*Table 18*). They are a safe alternative, provided that the patient has been properly measured for them, and they are more cosmetically acceptable to many people. They are not, however, particularly easy to put on. This problem can be overcome for many patients by supplying them with a dressing aid (*Figure 31*). Some manufacturers supply a silk half-sock to help the stocking to slide over the foot on application. The sock is removed by gently pulling it from the ends of the toes. Full length stockings are required in only a few circumstances, when treating patients with severe post-phlebitic syndrome, or lymphoedema with swelling in the thigh. Generally, below-knee stockings are all that is required, and as they are easier to apply than full length hosiery, compliance is likely to be better.

Figure 29a–f. Applying a bandage in a spiral.

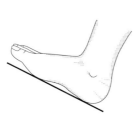

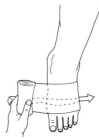

Figure 29a. Position the foot in a comfortable position, at a right angle to the leg.

Figure 29b. Begin by making 2 anchoring turns around the foot. Be sure to include the base of the toes.

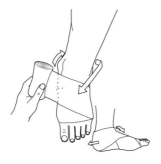

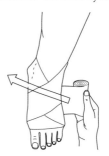

Figure 29c. Next take a high turn above the heel.

Figure 29d. Then fill the base of the foot with a low turn. From here, the bandage can be applied in a spiral as in this figure, or in a figure of eight (Figure 30).

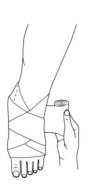

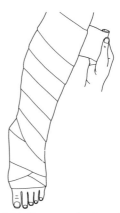

Figure 29e. Apply the bandage in a spiral, ensuring there is a 50% overlap.

Figure 29f. Ensure the bandage is applied right up to the tibial tuberosity.

Figure 30a–c. Applying a bandage in a figure of eight. To start the bandage complete steps a to d as shown in Figure 29.

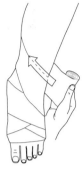 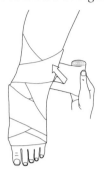 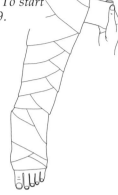

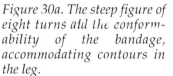

Figure 30a. The steep figure of eight turns and the conformability of the bandage, accommodating contours in the leg.

Figure 30b. Maintain these turns.

Figure 30c. Finish the bandaging at just below the knee.

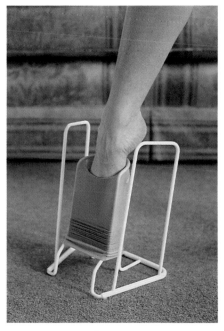 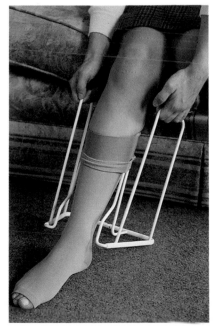

Figure 31a, b. A dressing aid such as Valet (by Medi) can solve the often difficult problem of putting on a compression stocking.

Compression stockings give graduated compression, with the greatest pressure exerted at the ankle, and are graded into three classes according to the compression they exert at the ankle:

- *Class I (14–17 mmHg)* Light compression, used to treat mild, early varicose veins.
- *Class II (18–24 mmHg)* Medium compression, for more serious varicosities, for patients who have had acute deep vein thrombosis, for the treatment of venous ulceration and for venous ulcer prevention.
- *Class III (25–35 mmHg)* Strong compression, for severe chronic venous hypertension, severe varicose veins, and ulcer prevention and treatment in patients with very large diameter calves.

Stockings are unlikely to be suitable for patients where high volumes of exudate are being produced. Once the quantity of exudate has been reduced, through good compression bandaging and a number of self-help measures (Section 4.7 and Chapter 5), stockings may then be a suitable option.

Although the initial cost of compression stockings is quite high, the cost over time is probably comparable with the cost of bandages for most patients.

4.1.7 *Intermittent compression therapy*

Intermittent pneumatic compression (IPC), sometimes referred to as sequential compression therapy (SCT), or sequential gradient pneumatic compression, is the therapeutic application of a controlled external pressure cycle on a limb using compressed air, which intermittently inflates a specially designed garment fitted to the limb (*Figure 32*). The effect of IPC is to improve venous return of blood to the heart from the peripheries, reduce oedema, and improve tissue oxygen perfusion. It is especially useful in patients with poor mobility, who are restricted in the extent to which they can aid venous return naturally through walking and other forms of exercise (Section 4.7.2).

Intermittent pneumatic compression has been used successfully in the management of:

- Chronic venous hypertension.
- Lymphoedema of the leg or arm.
- Oedema resulting from sporting injuries or a cerebrovascular accident.
- Deep vein thrombosis prophylaxis.

It has also been shown to enhance venous ulcer healing (Coleridge Smith *et al.*, 1990). Cornwall (1991) recommends treatment for a minimum period of two hours, twice a day for at least 6 weeks. After each treatment, graduated support stockings should be reapplied to maintain the reduction in oedema. Hazarika and Wright (1981) suggest that many elderly people living alone will require a great deal of support to overcome their fear of the electrical equipment (the air pump). Encouraging compliance with any regime, whether bandages, stockings or IPC, is especially important in the early stages, until the patient feels comfortable, confident and competent with it. There are anecdotal reports that once patients have begun to experience the benefits of IPC, and have become accustomed to fitting it in to their daily routine, they are reluctant to part with the equipment once the therapeutic need for it is over. For those who are afraid of the discomfort of compression, IPC is patient-friendly, because initial therapy can be for very short periods of low pressure, under the control of the patient. It is, of course, of limited value when there is also considerable oedema above the level of the IPC sleeve.

IPC is *contraindicated* in patients with:

- A deep vein thrombosis.
- Severe arteriosclerosis.
- Oedema due to congestive cardiac failure.
- Severe leg deformity.
- Local gangrene.

IPC is an adjunct to other therapies. Maximising mobility through exercise is essential, especially once the oedema is controlled, and no time should be lost between ceasing to apply IPC and the application of graduated compression bandages or stockings.

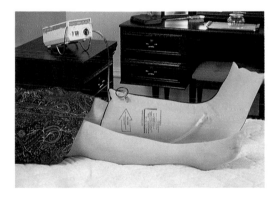

Figure 32. Intermittent pneumatic compression in use. (Huntleigh Technology, 1989)

4.1.8 Preventing and managing the recurrence of venous ulcers

The recurrence rate for leg ulceration is very high (Section 1.1). The self-help advice given in Section 4.7, and Chapter 5 (Appendices 5.2 and 5.3) should go some way to improving the circulation in the lower leg. The patient should be advised to take particular care to avoid knocking the leg, but should not be discouraged from going into public places where such trauma is most likely to occur. Social isolation can be one of the biggest problems for patients with recurrent ulcers. As with diabetic patients, extremes of temperature should be avoided, and garters and tight corsets which restrict blood circulation in the legs and feet should not be worn.

For patients with venous ulcers, wearing compression hosiery (*Figure 33*), even after the ulcer has healed, is one way of preventing recurrence. For some patients, surgery, such as saphenous vein ligation and stripping, or injection sclerotherapy for isolated varices, may be beneficial (Negus, 1991b).

A patient presenting with recurrent ulceration should be *reassessed* (Chapter 3) on *each* recurrence to determine whether there is any significant new pathology. A patient who presents at first with a venous ulcer may in time go on to develop significant arterial occlusion due to atherosclerosis which could contraindicate the use of compression therapy. The results of this assessment will determine the approach to management.

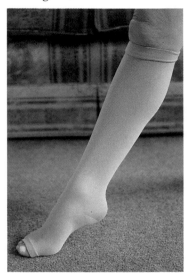

Figure 33. A class II compression stocking.

4.2   Management of arterial ulcers

The prognosis for an elderly patient with an arterial ulcer is much less hopeful than that for a patient with a venous ulcer properly treated, unless the underlying arterial problem is relatively local and is amenable to surgery. Where there are generalised arterial problems, such as arteritis, associated with rheumatoid arthritis, or micro-angiopathy, associated with diabetes mellitus, the treatment will be the doctor's responsibility. Vasodilator drugs are of questionable benefit, and even symptomatic relief of the effects of ischaemia is hard to achieve in some patients. The nurse's responsibility will be confined to symptom relief, local wound management (Section 4.6) and patient education (Chapter 5). The value of good nursing care in improving the patient's quality of life should not be underestimated.

Patients should be encouraged to mobilise to the limit of their capabilities, to stop smoking, to keep warm, to reduce weight, if overweight, and to eat a nutritious diet (Section 4.7).

The surgical management of arterial problems in the ulcerated limb is described by Negus (1991c). Thorough vascular assessment is required in order to determine the location and extent of atherosclerotic occlusion of the more major arteries, and the presence or absence of small vessel disease.

Compression bandaging should NOT be applied, as severe damage to the leg can result (*Figures 22, 34*).

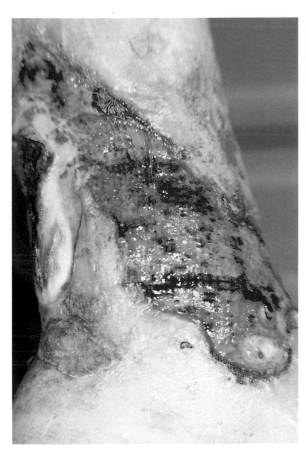

Figure 34. A deep arterial ulcer with exposure of the Achilles tendon. The ulcer developed from a minor skin lesion following the application of an elastic bandage.
(Ruckley, 1988)

4.3   Management of mixed aetiology ulcers

Where the underlying cause of the ulcer appears to be a *combination* of chronic venous hypertension and poor peripheral arterial circulation, it is the degree of *arterial* insufficiency which will determine whether or not it is safe to apply compression. If the resting pressure index (RPI) is *less than 0.8, no compression* should be applied unless under careful medical supervision (*Table 23*). If the RPI is 0.8–0.85, the patient may tolerate only light compression, such as a paste bandage with a light support bandage (Section 4.1.4 and *Table 19*). Patients vary widely in their tolerance of compression, and this, together with the RPI and a number of other factors, such as where, when, and by whom the bandage will be changed will determine the final regime selected.

Where there is significant peripheral arterial impairment, the doctor may at first decide to treat the arterial insufficiency conservatively. If vascular surgery is required, arterial bypass surgery is normally performed before venous surgery, to facilitate healing of the incisions created in the latter procedure. Ideally, the ulcer should be healed before vascular surgery is undertaken, but this may not be possible in cases of severe chronic venous hypertension, where compression therapy is contraindicated due to concurrent arterial disease. Angioplasty is being used increasingly to improve the arterial status sufficiently for the patient to receive compression for the venous component of the ulceration.

4.4   Management of ulcers associated with rheumatoid arthritis

The management of a patient with rheumatoid arthritis who has an ulcer on the lower limb depends very much on the underlying cause of the ulcer (Section 2.3). If the cause is primarily chronic venous hypertension then graduated compression therapy is required (Section 4.1). However, Negus (1991a) emphasises the importance of excluding arterial disease in these patients, when a very different set of treatment principles would apply (Section 4.2). Some factors of particular relevance to ulcer healing in any patient with rheumatoid arthritis are considered here.

The first is that deformity and disability in these patients increase the risk of traumatic injury. Many patients are on high dose steroid therapy which can have cutaneous effects, making the skin more susceptible to trauma and impairing some aspects of healing. The cutaneous manifestations of rheumatoid arthritis and the cutaneous complications of various treatments are described by Dunne and Robertson (1992).

The likelihood of delayed healing is increased in patients who are malnourished. Malnutrition is a common problem for people with rheumatoid arthritis, who may have a poor appetite. Furthermore, rheumatoid patients are more susceptible to infection. If they have vasculitis then this can lead to local ischaemia which also impairs healing.

The self-help measures described in Section 4.7 and Chapter 5 may pose particular problems where the person is severely disabled by arthritis and the active and ongoing cooperation of a member of the same household may be of crucial importance in facilitating compliance with treatment. Regular ankle and foot exercises are important, as with venous ulcers (Appendices 5.2 and 5.3). Particular attention should be paid to reducing pressure over high risk sites such as the heels when in bed, and to preventing even the most minor traumatic injuries. The skin should be kept supple and cracks treated with emollients. Special footwear may be required. Oedema may become an intractable problem for people with coexisting peripheral vascular disease who cannot tolerate limb elevation or any form of compression. Not surprisingly, perhaps, the success rate for skin grafting is poor (Pun *et al.*, 1990).

4.5   Management of the diabetic foot

The long-term management of diabetic patients, and the prevention of complications, is challenging. It requires a coordinated, multidisciplinary, team approach, which involves the physician, specialist diabetic nurse, chiropodist, and orthotist, and in some cases the vascular and orthopaedic surgeon. Above all, it requires informed patient cooperation.

Diabetic foot ulcers usually result from the triad of:

- Peripheral neuropathy (the insensate foot).
- Peripheral vascular insufficiency (ischaemia).
- Infection (Section 2.4).

According to Levin (1988), management of diabetic foot ulcers requires aggressive treatment. In the short term, this involves:

- Radical local debridement, leaving only healthy tissue.
- Systemic antibiotic therapy to combat infection, following antibiotic sensitivity testing.
- Diabetic control, which, among other effects, optimises efficiency of the immune system.
- Non-weight-bearing for plantar ulcers.

Appropriate wound dressing selection (Section 4.6.2) is important, but is merely an adjunct to the above therapies. Having stated this, the application of inappropriate topical agents can considerably worsen an already dire situation. If an ulcer is refractory to all treatment, the physician may request an X-ray to exclude the possibilities of osteomyelitis, or a retained foreign body that the patient does not feel.

Feet should be kept dry. Soaking the feet causes maceration between the toes and increases the risk of infection. Attention should also be given to rehydrating dry skin around the ulcer and over the lower leg with emollients.

For some patients, it is possible to improve the peripheral circulation through vascular bypass surgery, percutaneous angioplasty, laser treatment and the use of haemorrheologic agents, such as oxpentifylline (Trental), which improves red cell flexibility and blood flow. The combination of endovascular revascularisation, growth factor therapy, and comprehensive wound-care protocols can lead to very high limb-salvage rates in specialist centres (Bild et al. 1989; Knighton et al. 1990). However, prevention is infinitely preferable to cure. Some risk factors for peripheral vascular disease in diabetic patients are not treatable, such as age and the duration of the diabetes, but many risk factors are amenable to change, such as smoking, hypertension, hyperlipidaemia, hyperglycaemia, and obesity. Encouraging a diabetic patient to give up smoking and comply with dietary advice can significantly reduce many long-term complications. The nurse has a special part to play in reinforcing the advice given to patients (Chapter 5), as well as in local wound management (Section 4.6).

Patient education is, in fact, the key to preventing foot ulceration. All patients should receive special instruction in foot care (see Appendix 5.1), and their feet should be inspected at every routine outpatient visit, when this instruction should be reinforced. They should be encouraged to report foot problems as soon as they occur, however minor they appear to be. The chiropodist should trim the patient's toe nails, and treat calluses and other local foot problems. Local remedies applied by the patient are often the forerunners to serious foot problems.

Patients should be assessed for the need for special footwear to reduce pressure over bony prominences. Extra-depth shoes can be designed to accommodate clawed toes, and insoles can be made to reduce plantar pressures (Coleman, 1988). Total contact casting may be required for the management of diabetic neuropathic ulcers (Sinacore, 1988). Lightweight walking casts are described by Jones (1991). An orthopaedic scooter, as an energy saving aid for assisted ambulation, can give patients great freedom on level surfaces and can, in many situations, liberate the patient who must not weight-bear from crutches (Roberts and Carnes, 1990).

There are many conditions besides diabetes mellitus that can lead to poor peripheral arterial circulation in the legs and feet, including Buerger's disease, Raynaud's disease, and atherosclerosis. For further guidance on the management of arterial ulcers in the foot and leg, refer back to Section 4.2.

Diabetic patients can develop ulcers due to chronic venous hypertension in the absence of any history, clinical signs or symptoms of peripheral vascular disease or peripheral neuropathy. Compression should, however, always be applied with caution and under strict medical supervision.

4.6 Creating the optimum local environment for healing

4.6.0 Introduction

There is no doubt that correcting the *underlying cause* of an ulcer, where possible, is the first priority of leg ulcer management. There is some debate surrounding the relative importance and contribution of dressings to overall healing rates in patients with ulcers of vascular aetiology (Blair *et al.*, 1988; Moffatt *et al.*, 1992). However, it is important that dressings and other topical agents that are used do no harm, and are capable of contributing to the creation of optimum local conditions at the wound site. Adverse local conditions that may delay healing include infection, local dehydration, and the presence of dead or devitalized tissue, excess slough and excess exudate. Priorities in wound management, and the selection of the most appropriate primary wound dressing to overcome these problems, are discussed in Section 4.6.2. Other local treatment options, described below, include the use of ultrasound (Section 4.6.3), skin grafting (Section 4.6.4), the use of growth factors, keratinocyte autografts, and pharmacological agents (Section 4.6.5).

Creating the optimum local environment for healing begins with cleansing the whole leg.

4.6.1 Cleansing the leg

Before applying any kind of dressing to an ulcer, it is important to render the whole of the lower leg 'socially clean'. One way to do this is to immerse the leg in a deep plastic bowl lined with a disposable polythene bag, and half filled with lukewarm tap water. This helps to remove debris from the ulcer and the surrounding skin, and is comforting for the patient, especially if the leg has been encased in a multilayer bandage regimen for the previous week. The leg can be gently dried with soft disposable paper, and the bowl surface disinfected in accordance with the local infection control policy.

In the past, special precautions have been recommended where a wound was known to be infected with a virulent micro-organism, in order to reduce both the risk of contaminating the physical environment, and the risk of cross infection. If a patient was known to be infected with the Hepatitis B virus or with HIV (Human Immunodeficiency Virus), *barrier precautions* would be implemented to avoid contact with blood and body fluids. Most individuals infected with HIV are, however, unaware of their infection, and a new concept of infection control has emerged which is based on the proposition that *all clients are potentially infected*. This requires the adoption of *universal precautions* in clinical nursing practice.

Comprehensive infection control guidelines have been published both in the UK and the United States (Departments of Health, 1990; Centers for Disease Control, 1988). Specific and detailed infection control practice points, relevant to the nursing care of all patients in a variety of situations, are beyond the scope of this book but they are excellently summarised by Pratt (1992), based on the Departments of Health (1990) guidelines. Special attention should be paid to hand washing, and to the disposal of sharps and all contaminated materials. *Latex gloves* and a plastic apron should be worn by nurses for their own protection, and to prevent cross infection.

It is very important that practitioners remain clinically and professionally up to date on this important issue of public health, and adhere very strictly to the infection control policies laid down in their own Unit. Methods of safe disposal of contaminated materials in the *home* should be included in any infection control policy.

After cleansing, the ulcer can then be traced (*Figure 25*) before a dressing is applied.

4.6.2   Wound dressing selection

4.6.2.0   Aims and priorities The aims of local wound management are:

- To remove actual and potential causes of delayed healing.
- To create the optimum local environment for vascular and connective tissue reconstruction and epithelialisation.
- To protect the individual from further physiological damage.
- To relieve pain.

Priorities are essentially the same, whatever the wound, namely:

- Controlling bleeding (haemostasis).
- Removing foreign bodies.
- Managing clinical infection.
- Removing dead and devitalized tissue, thick slough and pus.
- Providing the optimum temperature, humidity and pH for the cells involved in the healing processes.
- Protecting the wound from further trauma and from the entry of potentially pathogenic micro-organisms. This often necessitates covering the wound with a dressing.

Haemostasis is rarely a problem, although bleeding can occur if a dressing adheres and is carelessly removed. Temporary application of direct pressure and elevation is normally sufficient to control this. Alternatively, an alginate dressing with haemostatic properties may be used under a retention or compression bandage.

Methods of removing foreign bodies are reviewed by Morison (1992b). This is rarely a problem for patients with leg ulceration, the main exception being for diabetic patients with significant peripheral neuropathy. These patients are unable to feel traumatically induced tissue damage. A retained foreign body, such as a nail or a splinter of metal, wood or glass, can lead to infection which, if not rapidly recognised and aggressively treated, can lead to the need for extensive surgical debridement or amputation (Section 4.5).

Much more commonly encountered problems for people with leg ulcers are described below, and include infection, the presence of necrotic tissue, excess slough and excess exudate. An algorithm (*Figure 35*) has been devised as an aid to teaching students the principal local treatment options. It is not intended to be fully comprehensive, or exclusive. As new products appear on the market and are proved to be clinically effective, they can be added. Where the weight of evidence suggests that a product may actually be harmful, it can be deleted. More detailed reviews of wound dressings, dressing selection and the value of a wound management policy are given by Morison (1992a), Thomas (1990) and Morgan (1990a, 1990b, 1992). Newer dressings are increasingly being systematically and rigorously assessed for efficacy, through randomised, controlled, clinical trials. To compensate for the large number of variables which could affect healing, besides the dressing, large numbers of patients are often required. Deciding on the end point in clinical trials is a vexed question. There is a strong argument for the approach which regards time to complete healing as the most appropriate end point. When reading research reports on dressing efficacy, special attention should be paid to the study design and the interpretation of results.

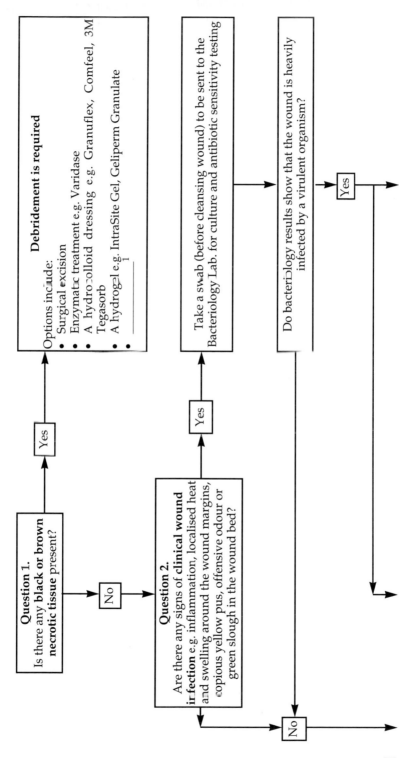

Figure 35. Which wound care product? Deciding priorities in the local management of open wounds, e.g. leg ulcers, diabetic foot ulcers, pressure sores, and fungating wounds.
Note: The sequence of the dressings for each indication is in alphabetical order by dressing type; dressings are NOT sequenced according

Question 1.
Is there any **black or brown necrotic tissue** present?

Yes

Debridement is required

Options include:
- Surgical excision
- Enzymatic treatment e.g. Varidase
- A hydrocolloid dressing e.g. Granuflex, Comfeel, 3M
- Tegasorb
- A hydrogel e.g. IntraSite Gel, Geliperm Granulate
- •

No

Question 2.
Are there any signs of **clinical wound infection** e.g. inflammation, localised heat and swelling around the wound margins, copious yellow pus, offensive odour or green slough in the wound bed?

Yes

Take a swab (before cleansing wound) to be sent to the Bacteriology Lab. for culture and antibiotic sensitivity testing

No

Do bacteriology results show that the wound is heavily infected by a virulent organism?

Yes

Superficial open wounds

If the wound is heavily contaminated or the patient is very debilitated, consider the use of:

- An activated charcoal dressing e.g. Actisorb Plus, Carbonet, Kaltocarb, Lyofoam C, OR
- An alginate sheet dressing e.g. Sorbsan, Kaltostat, (or Kaltostat Fortex if copious exudate) or Tegagel (changed daily and used in conjunction with systemic antibiotics), OR
- A topical antimicrobial agent, incorporated into a non-adherent dressing e.g. Bactigras, Chlorhexitulle, Inadine, OR
- A dressing containing Cadexomer iodine e.g. Iodosorb, Iodoflex[2], OR
- Flamazine cream (particularly for Gram-negative organisms e.g. *Pseudomonas sp.*), OR
- A foam dressing e.g. Lyofoam (in conjunction with systemic antibiotics), OR
- A hydrogel, e.g. Geliperm Granulate

1

Avoid use of topical antibiotics wherever possible.

Wound extending into dermis or deeper

Consider the use of:

- An activated charcoal dressing e.g. Actisorb Plus, Carbonet, Kaltocarb, Lyofoam C, OR
- An alginate rope or ribbon e.g. Kaltostat Cavity Dressing (changed daily and used in conjunction with systemic antibiotics), OR
- A bead dressing containing cadexomer iodine e.g. Iodosorb, Iodoflex[2], OR
- An enzymatic preparation e.g. Varidase to liquefy pus and break down excess slough, OR
- A hydrogel e.g. Geliperm Granulate, OR
- A polysaccharide bead dressing e.g. Debrisan, OR
- Sugar paste

In cases of severe local infection a systemic antibiotic may be required. Surgical excision of devitalized tissue may be necessary in extreme cases. Where anaerobic infection is a problem in fungating malodorous tumours, an amorphous hydrogel containing metranidazole, e.g. Metrotop, should be considered.

1

Desloughing is necessary.

Options include:

- Enzymatic treatment e.g. Varidase
- Hydrocolloid dressing e.g. Granuflex, Comfeel, 3M Tegasorb
- Hydrogel e.g. IntraSite Gel, Geliperm Granulate
- Polysaccharide beads or paste e.g. Debrisan, Iodosorb, Iodoflex[2], Dermaproof.

1

Question 3.
Is there excess **yellowish/grey/cream-coloured slough** present?

Yes

No

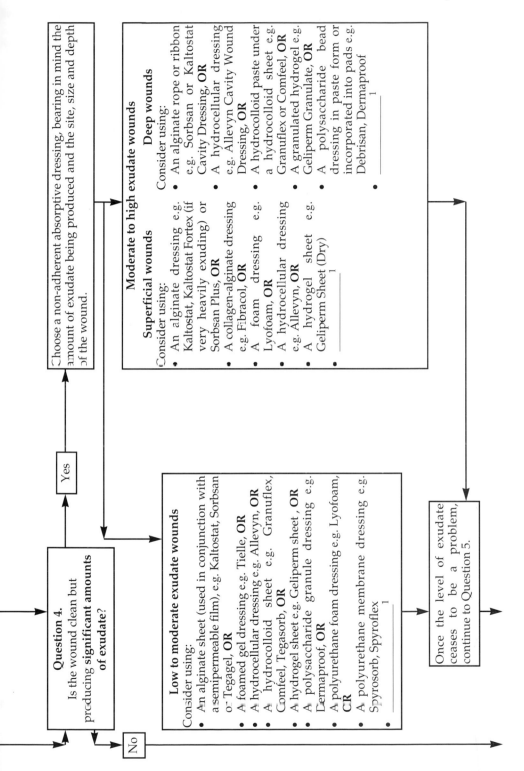

Question 4.
Is the wound clean but producing **significant amounts of exudate?**

Yes

No

Choose a non-adherent absorptive dressing, bearing in mind the amount of exudate being produced and the site, size and depth of the wound.

Moderate to high exudate wounds

Superficial wounds

Consider using:

- An alginate dressing e.g. Kaltostat, Kaltostat Fortex (if very heavily exuding) or Sorbsan Plus, **OR**
- A collagen-alginate dressing e.g. Fibracol, **OR**
- A foam dressing e.g. Lyofoam, **OR**
- A hydrocellular dressing e.g. Allevyn, **OR**
- A hydrogel sheet e.g. Geliperm Sheet (Dry)
- [1]

Deep wounds

Consider using:

- An alginate rope or ribbon e.g. Sorbsan or Kaltostat Cavity Dressing, **OR**
- A hydrocellular dressing e.g. Allevyn Cavity Wound Dressing, **OR**
- A hydrocolloid paste under a hydrocolloid sheet e.g. Granuflex or Comfeel, **OR**
- A granulated hydrogel e.g. Geliperm Granulate, **OR**
- A polysaccharide bead dressing in paste form or incorporated into pads e.g. Debrisan, Dermaproof
- [1]

Low to moderate exudate wounds

Consider using:

- An alginate sheet (used in conjunction with a semipermeable film), e.g. Kaltostat, Sorbsan o⁻Tegagel, **OR**
- A foamed gel dressing e.g. Tielle, **OR**
- A hydrocellular dressing e.g. Allevyn, **OR**
- A hydrocolloid sheet e.g. Granuflex, Comfeel, Tegasorb, **OR**
- A hydrogel sheet e.g. Geliperm sheet, **OR**
- A polysaccharide granule dressing e.g. Dermaproof, **OR**
- A polyurethane foam dressing e.g. Lyofoam, **OR**
- A polyurethane membrane dressing e.g. Spyrosorb, Spyroflex
- [1]

Once the level of exudate ceases to be a problem, continue to Question 5.

79

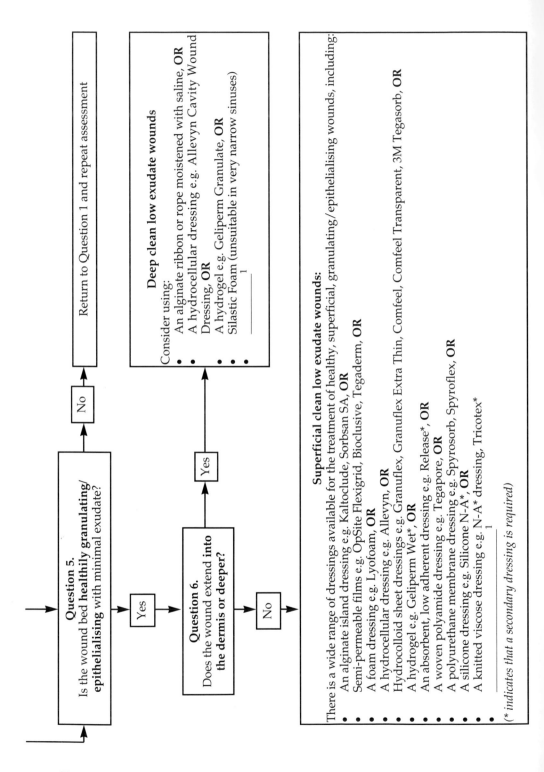

Question 5.
Is the wound bed **healthily granulating/ epithelialising** with minimal exudate?

No → Return to Question 1 and repeat assessment

Yes ↓

Question 6.
Does the wound extend into **the dermis or deeper?**

Yes → **Deep clean low exudate wounds**

Consider using:
• An alginate ribbon or rope moistened with saline, **OR**
• A hydrocellular dressing e.g. Allevyn Cavity Wound Dressing, **OR**
• A hydrogel e.g. Geliperm Granulate, **OR**
• Silastic Foam (unsuitable in very narrow sinuses)
1

No ↓

Superficial clean low exudate wounds:
There is a wide range of dressings available for the treatment of healthy, superficial, granulating/epithelialising wounds, including:
• An alginate island dressing e.g. Kaltoclude, Sorbsan SA, **OR**
• Semi-permeable films e.g. OpSite Flexigrid, Bioclusive, Tegaderm, **OR**
• A foam dressing e.g. Lyofoam, **OR**
• A hydrocellular dressing e.g. Allevyn, **OR**
• Hydrocolloid sheet dressings e.g. Granuflex, Granuflex Extra Thin, Comfeel, Comfeel Transparent, 3M Tegasorb, **OR**
• A hydrogel e.g. Geliperm Wet*, **OR**
• An absorbent, low adherent dressing e.g. Release*, **OR**
• A woven polyamide dressing e.g. Tegapore, **OR**
• A polyurethane membrane dressing e.g. Spyrosorb, Spyroflex, **OR**
• A silicone dressing e.g. Silicone N-A*, **OR**
• A knitted viscose dressing e.g. N-A* dressing, Tricotex*
1

(* *indicates that a secondary dressing is required*)

Notes:
[1] The product examples quoted in this algorithm are not intended to be regarded as an exhaustive or exclusive list of options. As new products become available and are proved to be effective, users may insert them in the appropriate spaces provided.
[2] Iodoflex (cadexomer iodine paste) is indicated for leg ulcers only (which includes venous, arterial, diabetic and foot ulcers).

This updated algorithm has been devised to aid nurses in deciding the most appropriate dressing for the local management of open wounds such as leg ulcers, diabetic foot ulcers, pressure sores and fungating wounds. The algorithm is a guide only. It is not intended to be fully comprehensive or exclusive. As new products appear on the market and are proved to be effective, they can be added in the space provided at the foot of each box.

In addition to the nature of the wound bed, many other factors should be considered before a dressing is selected, including:

- The site of the wound and ease, or otherwise, of applying the dressing
- The size of the wound
- The frequency of dressing changes required
- Comfort and cosmetic considerations
- Where and by whom the dressing will be changed
- The availability of the dressing in the size required – not all dressings are available to patients whose wounds are being managed in the community, and where a dressing is available on the Community Drug Tariff, it may not be available in all sizes.

Where all other considerations are equal, choose the cheapest dressing.

Before using any wound care product for the first time, ALWAYS consult the manufacturer's recommendations, contraindications, precautions and warnings. This information can change, so it is worth re-reading the manufacturer's instructions at frequent intervals. For 'prescription only' wound care products the relevant product data sheets MUST first be consulted prior to use.

If there is still any doubt about the suitability of any dressing , the patient's doctor should be consulted and further advice obtained from the local pharmacist.

It is particularly helpful when a health authority or unit has developed a wound care management policy (Morgan, 1990a, b). Whether or not a hospital has a list of recommended wound care products, the individual prescriber still has the final responsibility when it comes to dressing selection.

Further guidance on dressing selection, choice of cleansing solutions, the underlying principles of wound healing and the management of a wide variety of wounds is given in Morison (1992a).

81

4.6.2.1 Removing necrotic tissue The presence of dead or devitalized tissue in the wound bed may delay healing and make clinical infection more likely (*Figure 36*). The best method for treating this problem depends upon the nature of the necrotic tissue and the degree of debility of the patient. The necrotic tissue may be present in several forms, such as hard black eschar, and slough.

The main treatment options are:

- *Surgical debridement* This is the quickest method and results in a wound bed of healthy tissue. It can sometimes be performed under a local anaesthetic but may not be suitable for severely debilitated patients.
- *A hydrocolloid dressing or a hydrogel* These dressings help to create a local environment which encourages the body's natural debridement processes.
- *Enzymatic treatment (Figures 36, 37).*

The *hypochlorites* have been used in the past as debriding agents for the treatment of soft necrotic tissue, such as thick slough. However, they are quickly deactivated by body fluids and by the very waste products that they are likely to encounter, such as pus. Their use is *not recommended*, especially as there are much safer and more effective alternatives available today.

Whichever method of debridement is finally selected, **the manufacturer's recommendations should be consulted** concerning methods of application and removal, precautions, and any contraindications. More research is required to determine the most effective methods of debridement for different types of necrotic tissue in different clinical situations.

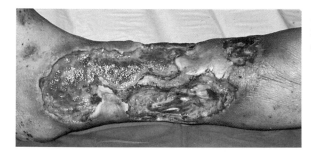

Figure 36. An extensive necrotic ulcer in an elderly diabetic patient.

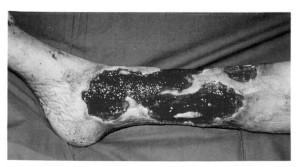

Figure 37. The same ulcer 7 days after debridement with an enzymatic preparation.

4.6.2.2 Treating clinical infection Chronic open wounds can be heavily *colonised* by micro-organisms, including many potential pathogens, without showing any adverse tissue response (Eriksson *et al.*, 1984). A number of studies have shown that the presence of colonising micro-organisms does not delay healing. Indeed, delayed healing is *more* likely if aggressive measures are taken to attempt to keep a chronic wound 'bacteria free'. A wound swab should therefore be sent to the bacteriology department for culture and antibiotic sensitivity testing only if the wound shows *clinical signs and symptoms of infection,* such as excess, malodorous exudate, erythema of the wound margins, or local pain and local oedema; or prior to grafting, to prevent graft loss due to infection which may not be clinically obvious.

If cellulitis is present (*Figure 38*), a *systemic antibiotic is normally prescribed*. The infection is present within the tissues, and can therefore not be reached using topically applied agents.

If a very virulent organism is isolated from a grossly infected open ulcer, with extensive tissue damage, the use of a *topical antiseptic,* such as cadexomer iodine, may be indicated (*Figures 39, 40*), in addition to systemic antibiotic therapy.

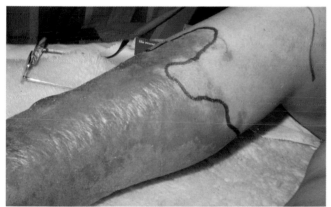

*Figure 38.
Cellulitis.
(Ruckley, 1988)*

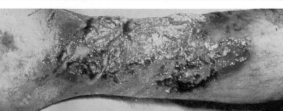

Figure 39. A grossly infected leg ulcer, with extensive necrotic tissue.

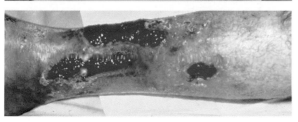

Figure 40. The same ulcer after treatment of the patient with a systemic antibiotic and the local application of a cadexomer iodine ointment.

There is some evidence that the injudicious, long-term use of topical antiseptics on chronic open wounds can actually *delay* healing. The evidence for and against the use of hypochlorites, and other chlorine-releasing solutions, such as Eusol, is reviewed by Brennan *et al.* (1986), Farrow and Toth (1991), Thomas (1991) and Moore (1992). Most of the studies reported have been done in animal models, and *in vitro*, rather than in humans.

The uses and potential pitfalls of a number of other popular cleansing agents and antiseptics are reviewed by Morison (1990).

A 'biological' alternative to the use of antiseptics in the local treatment of all but the most serious wound infections is to use an *enzyme based preparation*, which breaks down the *waste products* of infection, such as pus and slough, and creates a clean wound bed. The mainstay of treatment should still, however, be systemic antibiotics. These may need to be given intravenously in severe cases.

4.6.2.3 Managing malodorous ulcers Heavily infected leg ulcers can be very malodorous. This can be distressing for the patient, leading to self-imposed social isolation, loss of appetite and depression. Treating the infection that leads to the malodorous exudate is important (Section 4.6.2.2). The odour itself can be controlled in the short term by the use of an activated charcoal dressing. Wherever possible, dressings and bandages should be changed before 'strike through' of exudate has occurred. This reduces the risk of bacterial contamination through the wet dressing and the risk of the wound drying out and the dressing adhering.

4.6.2.4 Dressings for clean, deep ulcers Methods for dressing clean, deep ulcers producing some exudate include:

- *Alginate dressings.*
- *Hydrogels.*
- *Hydrocellular dressings.*
- *Polyurethane foam dressings.*
- *Polysaccharide granule dressings.*

If a wound is producing *copious volumes of exudate*, attempting to control this with a dressing is not enough. The skin surrounding the ulcer quickly becomes macerated, especially distally, and strike through of exudate increases the risk of wound infection. The oedema should be reduced, as described in Section 4.7.3, and then the level of exudate will lessen until a stage is reached when weekly dressing changes are sufficient. In the meantime, extra absorbent padding can be applied over the primary dressing and under the bandages.

4.6.2.5 Dressings for clean, shallow ulcers There are a number of primary dressings suitable for clean, shallow leg ulcers, whether they are venous or arterial in origin. These include:

- *Polyurethane membrane dressings.*
- *Woven polyamide dressings.*
- *Silicone dressings.*
- *Knitted viscose dressings.*
- *Polyurethane foam dressings.*
- *Hydrocellular dressings.*
- *Alginate dressings.*
- *Hydrocolloid sheet dressings.*

Some of the factors which will influence the choice of dressing are listed at the end of *Figure 35.*

4.6.2.6 Sensitivity to wound care products Sensitivity to components found in topical skin and wound preparations is a common phenomenon in patients with leg ulcers (Kulozik *et al.,* 1988). Signs and symptoms of a sensitivity reaction include marked erythema of the skin where the product has been in contact, aggravation of pre-existing eczematous conditions, and itching (*Figure 41*).

The most common causes of sensitivity reactions include:

- *Topical antibiotics* (e.g. neomycin or Framycetin sulphate).
- *Bases of ointments* (e.g. lanolin).
- *Preservatives* (e.g. parabens).

Several proprietary antiseptics and antihistamine creams that patients buy and administer to themselves can also cause an adverse skin reaction. The paste bandages (*Table 22*) can cause sensitivity reactions in some patients. There is some evidence to suggest that the longer an ulcer has been open, the more skin and wound care products the patient is likely to be sensitive to.

If a sensitivity reaction does occur, use of the sensitising agent should be discontinued at once, and the event clearly documented in the patient's notes. A steroid cream may be prescribed by the doctor for application to the skin surrounding the ulcer. Allergy to steroids also occurs! Only the blandest of dressings should be applied to the wound itself.

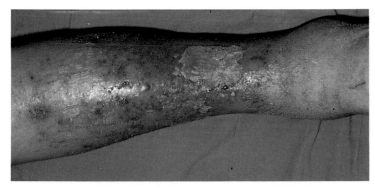

Figure 41. Contact dermatitis.

Patch testing can be helpful in identifying allergens (Cameron, 1990). Negative results should, however, be viewed with caution as late positive reactions can occur three weeks or more after the patch test (Paramsothy *et al.*, 1988). For more information on the dermatological aspects of ulcer management, the reader is referred to the texts listed in Further Reading at the end of this chapter. Many of these specialist texts are superbly illustrated.

4.6.3 *Ultrasound*

Several studies have suggested that ultrasound can promote healing in chronic wounds, and results in healed wounds with greater strength and elasticity. Callam *et al.* (1987) found that a once-weekly treatment with ultrasound was effective when used as an adjunct to compression therapy. The role of ultrasound in wound healing is reviewed by Dyson (1990).

4.6.4 *Skin grafting*

Most venous ulcers can be successfully treated using graduated compression bandaging or stockings. However, the healing of large venous ulcers may be accelerated by simple skin grafting methods, using either pinch or meshed split skin (Poskitt *et al.*, 1987; Moffatt and Oldroyd, 1989). Such methods can be performed even on outpatients taken as day cases, but greater success is likely to be attained with inpatient care. Before grafting is carried out, a period of bed rest is usually required to reduce oedema and promote the formation of healthy granulation tissue. The successful take of a graft requires a 'clean' wound bed, free from potential pathogens such as haemolytic streptococci and pseudomonads, and depends on the rapid development of a new blood supply. Grafts fail because of:

- *Inadequate blood supply in the recipient area.*
- *Haematoma*, which prevents vascular link up and increases the risk of infection.
- *Shearing forces*, which cause the graft to move, severing newly joined vessels.
- *Infection*.

In a healthy graft, capillary link-up is well under way by the third day, and within four days the graft is usually sufficiently stable to be safely handled if reasonable care is taken (McGregor, 1990).

A successful skin graft can give a new lease of life to a patient who has suffered from chronic ulceration for many years (Moody, 1984), but, in itself, is no guarantee that ulceration will not recur.

4.6.5 *Looking to the future*

There are some very exciting developments on the horizon in wound management. Several new approaches to promoting healing are currently being assessed, including the use of growth factors to accelerate healing (McKay and Leigh, 1991). Many growth factors have now been isolated, including:

- Epidermal growth factor (EGF).

- Platelet-derived growth factor (PDGF).
- Fibroblast growth factors (FGFs).
- Transforming growth factor-beta (TGF-β).

These growth factors have been reported to be highly potent agents in promoting healing in animal models, even in very low doses. They can now be manufactured in large quantities using recombinant DNA technology. Clinical trials in humans are well under way in many specialist centres, both in the USA and in the UK. However, many questions remain to be answered:

- At what stage in the healing process should each be used?
- Are there any adverse effects, and in what circumstances?
- Do the clinical benefits justify the costs involved?

Another exciting development is the culture of skin grafts in the laboratory from a patient's own cells (Phillips, 1988; Hancock and Leigh, 1989). The grafts are called keratinocyte autografts. Clinical trials have demonstrated that these grafts have major lifesaving potential in the management of patients with very extensive skin loss, such as that resulting from burns. They have also been used successfully to treat skin disorders such as epidermolysis bullosa, and chronic wounds such as leg ulcers. As with growth factors, the question of whether the clinical benefits justify the costs must be asked in relation to the treatment of leg ulcers where a range of very effective treatments already exists.

Much research is currently underway on the role of pharmacological agents in leg ulcer management. Most are aimed at improving the microcirculation in the limb and preventing lipodermatosclerosis. So far, these are adjuvant therapies. Two research studies and a review of the role of pharmacological agents are included in Further Reading.

4.7 Wider issues

4.7.1 Causes of delayed healing

The main cause of delayed healing in leg ulcers is:

FAILURE TO IDENTIFY AND TREAT THE UNDERLYING CAUSE OF THE ULCER

Other causes of delayed healing include local wound infection (Section 4.6.2.2), sensitivity to wound care products (Section 4.6.2.6), and a number of *general patient factors* (*Figure 27*). Factors particularly significant for patients with leg ulcers include:

- Restricted mobility.
- Oedema in the limb.
- Malnutrition.
- Psychosocial problems.

4.7.2 Restricted mobility

Poor mobility is a very common problem for elderly patients with leg ulcers, whether due to joint stiffness, neuromuscular disorders, obesity, or respiratory problems. It is essential to improve mobility in patients with any type of leg ulcer. This aids venous return by activating the calf muscle pump, as well as reducing the risk of other problems associated with prolonged immobility, such as chest infections and deep vein thromboses.

Patients should be encouraged to mobilise to the limits of their ability. For a patient with advanced arterial disease the limit may be 100–200 yards or metres, or even less. By contrast, many patients with venous ulcers are capable of walking 2–3 miles (3–5 km) per day, and should be encouraged to do so. This is the ideal, but may be unattainable for many elderly patients, especially if their poor mobility is accompanied by chronic respiratory problems. It is in circumstances such as these that intermittent pneumatic compression may be particularly helpful in reducing oedema in patients with venous ulcers (Section 4.1.7).

The *physiotherapist* may need to be involved if the patient has restricted ankle movements or other musculoskeletal problems. Housebound patients can be encouraged to walk on the spot for a few minutes every hour. Prolonged standing in one place should be avoided. Washing up and ironing can be done sitting down if chairs of suitable height are available. Chair-bound patients can be taught ankle extension, flexion and rotation exercises by the physiotherapist or nurse (Appendix 5.3).

4.7.3 Peripheral oedema

There are many causes of peripheral oedema, including cardiac failure, liver disease, venous or lymphatic disease, and malnutrition (Reilly and Wolfe, 1991). Peripheral oedema in a dependent limb can also be encountered in a patient with hemiparesis following a cerebrovascular accident. Identification by the doctor of the underlying cause of the oedema is important, as this will determine the treatment.

Whatever its cause, peripheral oedema in the lower limb delays healing by increasing the diffusion distance between blood capillaries and the tissues they serve. The tissues become starved of oxygen and nutrients, and metabolic waste products build up.

Improving mobility (Section 4.7.2) is one very important way of reducing oedema.

Elevation is always desirable when at rest, provided there is a good arterial supply. For patients with venous ulcers, sitting with the legs elevated *above the level of the hips* (Appendices 5.2 and 5.3) helps to reduce oedema by aiding venous return of blood to the heart. It is *not* sufficient to raise the legs a little above the ground by placing them on a low foot stool. Assessment of the home environment may be very helpful. The most suitable furniture may not be in the room in which the patient lives. The television may need to be repositioned in a more appropriate location to encourage compliance with leg elevation.

Most patients will benefit from sleeping with the *foot of the bed raised by about 9 inches* (23 cm). This aids venous return and can significantly reduce oedema overnight. However, sudden return of fluid to the heart caused by leg elevation can precipitate cardiac and/or respiratory failure in frail elderly patients. It is therefore advisable to check with the patient's physician that leg elevation is not contraindicated. It is unlikely to be tolerated in patients with poor arterial circulation, who often find it necessary to lower the affected limb below the heart to reduce ischaemic rest pain.

Severe oedema can be alleviated by bed rest, but prolonged bed rest causes problems of its own. Patients may be less mobile when they get up, with stiffened ankle and knee joints. They may develop a chest infection, or a deep vein thrombosis which could further damage the valves in their veins.

4.7.4 Malnutrition

As with all wounds, delayed healing is inevitable if the patient's diet is deficient in protein, calories, vitamins (such as A and C) and minerals (such as iron, zinc and copper).

Malnutrition is a common problem for the elderly for many reasons:

- Poverty.
- Difficulty in getting to the shops and in preparing food.
- Loss of interest in diet when living alone.
- Ill-fitting dentures.
- Specific gastrointestinal disorders involving malabsorption problems.

If malnutrition is suspected, a full patient assessment should be carried out by the *dietician* (Taylor and Goodinson–McLaren, 1992). If the diet is deficient in vitamins and minerals, overweight patients can be just as 'malnourished' as the obviously underweight patient. **The control of obesity can make a crucial contribution to ulcer healing** by reducing prolonged back pressure in the venous system, caused by deep vein obstruction in the pelvic area (*Figure 5*), as well as by enabling increased mobility.

Where the causes of malnutrition are largely social, the *district nurse, health visitor* or *social worker* can help to arrange meals on wheels, lunch club activities, etc.

4.7.5 Psychosocial issues

Many patients with leg ulcers are elderly, poor and alone. They welcome the visit of the community nurse treating their ulcer because of the social contact that it brings.

Much has been written about the 'social' ulcer. There is no doubt that some patients do not have a vested interest in their ulcer healing, but the proportion of patients who actually *interfere* with the ulcer in an attempt to delay healing is unknown.

Many patients who interfere with their bandages do so for very good reasons:

- The bandage may have been applied under *too much tension*, especially over the dorsum of the foot, causing considerable discomfort.

89

- The bandage may have slipped, causing a tight band of constriction, and pain over a bony prominence.
- A bulky bandage may be causing the patient problems with wearing ordinary footwear.

Prodding a knitting needle between the bandage and the leg may be the patient's solution to an intolerable itch, rather than a wilful attempt at undoing the nurse's good work.

The natural recurrence rate for leg ulceration is also high, especially if no measures are taken to prevent recurrence. An indication that the ulcer is factitious is the occurrence of an ulcer in a bizarre site or of an unusual appearance, but the more unusual causes of ulceration (Section 2.5) should be considered.

If, after exploring with the patient the reasons behind obvious tampering with bandages and dressings, a conscious attempt at self-inflicted injury is still suspected, the problem *must* be dealt with sympathetically. If the problem is one of loneliness, ways of improving the patient's social contacts should be explored with the district nurse, health visitor or social work department. If the patient is finding it increasingly difficult to cope alone at home, some form of day care may need to be considered. A 'well ulcer' clinic can be helpful to overcome the loss of social contacts once an ulcer has healed.

The patient's role in contributing to successful treatment should not be underestimated, and will be discussed in more detail in the next chapter.

Further reading

Compression therapy for venous ulcers

Blair, S.D., Wright, D.D.I., Backhouse, C.M., Riddle, E. & McCollum, C.N. (1988) Sustained compression and healing of chronic venous ulcers. *BMJ* **297**, 1159–1161.

Coleridge Smith, P., Sarin, S., Hasty, J. & Scurr, J.H. (1990) Sequential gradient pneumatic compression enhances venous ulcer healing: a randomised trial. *Surgery* **108**, 871–875.

Cornwall, J.V., Dore, C.J. & Lewis, J.D. (1987) Graduated compression and its relation to venous refilling time. *BMJ* **295**, 1087–1090.

Fentem, P.H. (1990) Defining the compression provided by hosiery and bandages. *Care: Science and Practice* **8(2)**, 53–55.

Ruckley, C.V. (1992) Treatment of venous ulceration – compression therapy. *Phlebology Supplement* **1**, 22–26

Sockalingham, S., Barbenel, J.C. & Queen, D. (1990) Ambulatory monitoring of the pressures beneath compression bandages. *Care: Science and Practice* **8(2)**, 75–79.

Thomas, S. (1990) Bandages and bandaging. *Nurs Stand* **4(39)**, 4–6.

Surgical management of venous disease

Negus, D. (1991) *Leg Ulcers: A Practical Approach to Management* Butterworth–Heinemann, Oxford.

Ruckley, C.V. (1988) *A Colour Atlas of Surgical Management of Venous Disease* Wolfe Medical Publications, London.

Diabetic foot ulcers

Boulton, A.J.M. (1988) The diabetic foot. *Med Clin North Am* **72(6)**, 1513–1530.

Harrelson, J.M. (1989) Management of the diabetic foot. *Orthop Clin North Am* **20(4)**, 605–619.

Levin, M.E. (1988) The diabetic foot: pathophysiology, evaluation and treatment. In: Levin, M.E. & O'Neal, L.W. (eds) *The diabetic foot* (4th edn) CV Mosby, St. Louis, pp. 1–50.

Robertson, J.C., Daunt, S.O'N. & Nur, M. (1986) Tissue viability – wound healing and the diabetic. *Practical Diabetes* **3**, 14–19.

Vasculitic ulcers

Cawley, M.I. (1987) Vasculitis and ulceration in rheumatic diseases of the foot. *Bailliere's Clin Rheumatol* **1(2)**, 315–333.

Conn, D.L. (ed) (1990) Vasculitic syndromes. *Rheum Dis Clin North Am* **16(2)** (whole issue, but see particularly pp. 269–292).

Physiology of wound healing and pathophysiology of non-healing

Forrester, J.C. (1988) Wound healing and fibrosis. In: Ledingham, I. & Mackay, C. (eds) *Textbook of surgical physiology*, (4th edn) Churchill Livingstone, Edinburgh, pp. 1–15.

Morison, M.J. (1992) The physiology of wound healing. In: Morison, M.J. *A Colour Guide to the Nursing Management of Wounds* Wolfe Publishing, London, pp. 1–21.

Niinikoski, J., Gottrup, F. & Hunt, T.K. (1991) The role of oxygen in wound repair. In: Janssen, H., Rooman, R. & Robertson, J.I.S. (eds) *Wound Healing* Wrightson Biomedical Publishing, Petersfield, pp. 165–174.

Ryan, T.J. (1991) Pathophysiology of non-healing chronic wounds: biochemical control of grip and stick. In: Janssen, H., Rooman, R. & Robertson, J.I.S. (eds) *Wound Healing* Wrightson Biomedical Publishing, Petersfield, pp. 127–135.

Wound dressings and dressing selection

Morgan, D.A. (1992) *Formulary of wound management products: a guide for health care staff* (5th edn) Media Medica, Chichester.

Morison, M.J. (1992) Priorities in wound management: which dressing? In: Morison, M.J. *A Colour Guide to the Nursing Management of Wounds* Wolfe Publishing, London, pp. 33–47.

Thomas, S. (1990) *Wound Management and Dressings* The Pharmaceutical Press, London.

Wiseman, D.M., Rovee, D.T. & Alvarez, O.M. (1992) Wound dressings: design and use. In: Cohen, I.K., Diegelmann, R.F. & Lindblad, W.J. (eds) *Wound Healing: Biomedical and Clinical Aspects*, WB Saunders, Philadelphia, pp. 562–580.

The role of pharmacological agents

Colgan, M., Dormandy, J.A., Jones, P.W., Schraibman, I.G., Shanik, D.G. & Young, R.A.L. (1990) Oxpentifylline treatment for venous ulcers of the leg. *BMJ* **300**, 972–975.

Negus, D. (1991) Pharmacological treatment of leg ulcers. In: Negus, D. *Leg Ulcers: a Practical Approach to Management.* Butterworth–Heinemann, Oxford, pp. 119–124.

Wright, D.D.I., Franks, P.J., Blair, S.D., Backhouse, C.M., Moffatt, C. & McCollum, C.N. (1991) Oxerutins in the prevention of recurrence in chronic venous ulceration: randomised controlled trial. *Br J Surg* **78**, 1269–1270.

Dermatological aspects

du Vivier, A. (1993) Skin manifestations of disordered circulation. In: du Vivier, A. *Atlas of Clinical Dermatology* (2nd edn) Gower Medical Publishing, London, Chapter 21.

Holgate, S.T. & Church, M.K. (1993) *Allergy* Gower Medical Publishing, London.

Jackson, W.F. & Cerio, R. (1988) *A Colour Atlas of Allergy* Wolfe Medical Publications, London.

Stone, L.A., Lindfield, E.M. & Robertson, S. (1989) *A Colour Atlas of Nursing Procedures in Skin Disorders* Wolfe Medical Publications, London.

Wilkinson, J.D. & Rycroft, R.J.G. (1992) Contact dermatitis. In: Champion, R.H., Burton, J.L. & Ebling, F.J.G. (eds) *Textbook of Dermatology.* Blackwell Scientific Publications, Oxford, pp. 611–715.

Wider issues: pain and nutrition

McCaffery, M. & Beebe, A. (1989) *Pain: Clinical Manual for Nursing Practice* C.V. Mosby, St. Louis.

McLaren, S.M.G. (1992) Nutrition and wound healing. *Journal of Wound Care* **1(3)** 45–55.

References

Bild, D.E., Selby, J.V. & Sinnock, P. (1989) Lower extremity amputation in people with diabetes: epidemiology and prevention. *Diab Care* **12**, 24–31.

Blair, S.D., Backhouse, C.M., Wright, D.D.I., Riddle, E. & McCollum, C.N. (1988) Do dressings influence the healing of chronic venous ulcers? *Phlebology* **3**, 129–134.

Brennan, S.S., Foster, M.E. & Leaper, D.J. (1986) Antiseptics toxicity in wounds healing by secondary intention. *J Hosp Infect* **8(3)**, 263–267.

Callam, M.J., Harper, D.R., Dale, J.J., Ruckley, C.V. & Prescott, R.J. (1987) A controlled trial of weekly ultrasound therapy in chronic leg ulceration. *Lancet* **ii**, 204–206.

Cameron, J. (1990) Patch testing for leg ulcer patients. *Nursing Times* **86(25)**, 63–64.

Centers for Disease Control (1988) Update: universal precautions for prevention of transmission of Human Immunodeficiency Virus, Hepatitis B Virus and other bloodborne pathogens in health care settings. *MMWR* **37** (24 June), 377–388.

Coleman, W.C. (1988) Footwear in a management program of injury prevention. In: Levin, M.E. & O'Neal, L.W. (eds) *The Diabetic Foot* (4th edn.) CV Mosby, St. Louis, pp. 293–309.

Coleridge Smith, P., Sarin, S., Hasty, J. & Scurr, J.H. (1990) Sequential gradient pneumatic compression enhances venous ulcer healing: a randomised trial. *Surgery* **108**, 871–875.

Cornwall, J. (1991) Managing venous leg ulcers. *Community Outlook* **May**, 36–38.

Departments of Health, (1990) *Guidance for clinical healthcare workers: protection against infection with HIV and hepatitis viruses, recommendations of the expert advisory group on AIDS* HMSO, London.

Dunne, C. & Robertson, J. (1992) Wound healing in rheumatoid arthritis. *Wound Management* **2(4)**, 13–14.

Dyson, M. (1990) Role of ultrasound in wound healing. In: Kloth, L.C. et al. (eds) *Wound Healing: Alternatives in Management*. FA Davis, Philadelphia 259–285

Eriksson, G., Ekland, A. & Kallings, L.O. (1984) The clinical significance of bacterial growth in venous leg ulcers. *Scand J Infect Dis* **16**, 175–180.

Farrow, S. & Toth, B. (1991) The place of Eusol in wound management. *Nurs Stand* **5(22)**, 25–27.

Hancock, K. & Leigh, I.M. (1989) Cultured keratinocytes and keratinocyte grafts. *BMJ* **299**, 1179–1180.

Hazarika, E.Z. & Wright, D.E. (1981) Chronic leg ulcers: the effect of pneumatic intermittent compression. *Practitioner* **225**, 189–192.

Jones, G.R. (1991) Walking casts: effective treatment for foot ulcers? *Practical Diabetes* **8(4)**, 131–132.

Knighton, D.R., Fylling, C.P. & Fiegel, V.D. et al. (1990) Amputation prevention in an independently reviewed at risk diabetic population using a comprehensive wound care protocol. *Am J Surg* **160**, 466–472.

Kulozik, M., Powell, S.M., Cherry, G. & Ryan, T.J. (1988) Contact sensitivity in community-based leg ulcer patients. *Clin Exp Dermatol* **13**, 82–84.

Levin, M.E. (1988) The diabetic foot: pathophysiology, evaluation and treatment. In: Levin, M.E. & O'Neal, L.W. (eds) *The Diabetic Foot* (4th edn) CV Mosby, St. Louis, pp. 1–50.

McGregor, I.A. (1990) *Fundamental Techniques of Plastic Surgery and their Surgical Applications* (8th edn) Churchill Livingstone, Edinburgh.

McKay, I.A. & Leigh, I.M. (1991) Epidermal cytokines and their roles in cutaneous wound healing. *Br J Dermatol* **124**, 513–518.

Moffatt, C. (1992) Compression bandaging – the state of the art. *Journal of Wound Care* **1(1)**, 45–50.

Moffatt, C.J., Franks, P.J., Oldroyd, M.I. & Greenhalgh, R.M. (1992) Randomised trial of an occlusive dressing in the treatment of chronic non-healing leg ulcers. *Phlebology* **7**, 105–107.

Moffatt, C.J. & Oldroyd, M. (1989) Pinch skin grafting: an extension of the role of the nurse specialist. *Primary Health Care* **7(7)**, 18–20.

Moody, M. (1984) A new lease of life. *Nursing Times* **July 4**, 46.

Moore, D. (1992) Hypochlorites: a review of the evidence. *Journal of Wound Care* **1(4)**, 44–53.

Morgan, D.A. (1990a) Development of a wound management policy: Part 1. *Pharm J* **244**, 295–297.

Morgan, D.A. (1990b) Development of a wound management policy: Part 2. *Pharm J* **244**, 358–359.

Morgan, D.A. (1992) *Formulary of Wound Management Products: a Guide for Health Care Staff* (5th edn) Media Medica, Chichester.

Morison, M.J. (1990) Wound cleansing – which solution? *Nurs Stand* **4(52) Suppl.** 4–6.

Morison, M.J. (1992a) *A Colour Guide to the Nursing Management of Wounds* Wolfe Publishing, London, pp. 33–47.

Morison, M.J. (1992b) Traumatic wounds. In Morison, M.J. *A Colour Guide to the Nursing Management of Wounds* Wolfe Publishing, London, pp. 186–203.

Negus, D. (1991a) *Leg Ulcers: A Practical Approach to Management* Butterworth–Heinemann, Oxford.

Negus, D. (1991b) Definitive treatment: prevention of recurrence of venous ulceration. In: Negus, D. *Leg Ulcers: A Practical Approach to Management* Butterworth–Heinemann, Oxford, pp. 125–148.

Negus, D. (1991c) The treatment of ischaemic and other leg ulcers; recurrent ulceration. In: Negus, D. *Leg Ulcers: A Practical Approach to Management* Butterworth–Heinemann, Oxford, pp. 149–155.

Paramsothy, Y., Collins, M. & Smith, G.M. (1988) Contact dermatitis in patients with leg ulcers: the prevalence of late positive reactions. *Contact Dermatitis* **18**, 30–36.

Phillips, T. (1988) Cultured skin grafts. *Arch Dermatol* **124**, 1035–1038.

Poskitt, K.R., Lloyd-Davies, E.R.V., James, A., Walton, J. & McCollum, C.N. (1987) Pinch grafting or porcine dermis in venous ulcers: a randomised clinical trial. *BMJ* **294**, 674–676

Pratt, R. (1992) *AIDS: A Strategy for Nursing Care* (3rd edn) Edward Arnold, London.

Pun, Y.L.W., Barraclough, D.R.E. & Muirden, K.D. (1990) Leg ulcers in rheumatoid arthritis. *Med J Aust* **153(10)**, 585–587.

Reilly, D.T. & Wolfe, J.H.N. (1991) The swollen leg. *BMJ* **303**, 1462–1465.

Roberts, P. & Carnes, S. (1990) The orthopaedic scooter: an energy-saving aid for assisted ambulation. *J Bone Joint Surg* **72**, 620–621.

Ruckley, C.V. (1988) *A Colour Atlas of Surgical Management of Venous Disease* Wolfe Medical Publications, London.

Sinacore, D.R. (1988) Total-contact casting in the treatment of diabetic neuropathic ulcers. In: Levin, M.E. & O'Neal, L.W, (eds) *The Diabetic Foot* (4th edn) CV Mosby, St. Louis, pp. 273–292.

Sockalingham, S., Barbenel, J.C. & Queen, D. (1990) Ambulatory monitoring of the pressures beneath compression bandages. *Care: Science and Practice* **8(2)**, 75–79.

Stone, L.A., Lindfield, E.M. & Robertson, S. (1989) *A Colour Atlas of Nursing Procedures in Skin Disorders* Wolfe Medical Publications, London.

Taylor, S. & Goodinson-McLaren, S. (1992) *Nutritional Support: A Team Approach* Wolfe Publishing, London.

Thomas, S. (1990) *Wound Management and Dressings* The Pharmaceutical Press, London.

Thomas, S. (1991) Evidence fails to justify use of hypochlorite. *Journal of Tissue Viability* **1(1)**, 9–10.

5.   Patient education

5.1   Why educate patients?

A very wide range of factors is now known to affect wound healing in any patient (*Figure* 27), and some factors are particularly significant for patients with a leg ulcer. Methods for reducing oedema, and improving mobility and nutritional status, were described in Section 1.7. All require active patient cooperation.

The extent to which *non-compliance* with professionally given advice occurs and delays healing is not known. In the community, ongoing supervision by the nurse can increase compliance, especially where the relationship between the nurse and the patient is perceived by the patient to be good. However, the patient must also believe that in the long term the treatment will be effective. Giving patients hope is part of the art of healing. Other factors which are thought to affect compliance include:

- The extent to which the patients understand what it is they are to do.
- The patient's perception of the severity of the condition.
- The presence or absence of pain.
- The amount of change required in the patient's lifestyle.
- The amount of inconvenience involved, offset against the perceived potential benefits.
- The complexity of the regimen that the patient is asked to undertake.

Teaching patients the self-help skills which they should practise for the rest of their lives to promote healing and prevent ulcer recurrence requires patience, skill, and an understanding of the individual and the individual's personal circumstances. It involves assessing the patient's personality and cognitive abilities, deciding on the level and amount of information that the person requires and when and how to impart it, and deciding how to evaluate whether the teaching is having the desired effect. It also involves positive reinforcement, appropriate to the individual, for any efforts that are made towards their own health promotion. Even a few words of praise can be very effective in encouraging persistence with self-help measures, as they show an appreciation for the efforts that the individual is making, and enhance the individual's self-esteem.

Providing accurate information is important. It is also important to verify that the patient has understood the information given, and knows how to apply it. However, information and understanding are not enough. Ultimately, a successful long-term outcome depends upon the success of the health educator in motivating patients to *take responsibility for their own health*, to the limit of their ability. This involves encouraging patients to change their behaviour in positive ways, to promote health and wellbeing. This is no easy task, especially when the behavioural changes required involve giving up long-held strategies, such as overeating and smoking, aimed at coping with the stresses of every day living. The importance of assessing the psychosocial factors that could affect compliance with treatment and healing was stressed in Chapter 3.

The patient's role in facilitating healing cannot be over-emphasised.

The first, and perhaps the most crucial step in bringing about positive behavioural change is to create a *therapeutic environment* which encourages the patient to *engage* in the learning process, and which motivates the patient to want to change unhelpful behaviour.

5.2 Creating a therapeutic environment for learning

The basis of effective education is *empathy* between the educator and the patient (Tschudin, 1991).

Empathy involves understanding a patient's feelings about a situation *from his or her perspective* and *communicating this understanding* in a way which indicates both awareness of, and respect for, the individual as a person, and acknowledges the individual's specific needs.

Disease and disability can involve threats not only to physical wellbeing but also to a person's self-image, social and occupational functioning, and emotional equilibrium (Weinman, 1982). The consequences of a wound for an individual will depend on many factors, including:

- The site and type of wound.
- The degree of functional disability.
- The visibility of scarring.
- The availability of social support.
- The level of economic independence.
- The person's personality and personal philosophy.
- The accuracy of the appraisal by the person of his or her prognosis.

The possible effects of a leg ulcer on the individual's quality of life were described in Section 1.6. They can be very far reaching, affecting the person's social life as well as physical functioning.

In a therapeutic relationship, patients are helped to understand where they are (the here and now) in relation to where they would like to be (the goal) (*Figure 42*). Effective *patient-centred communication* is a prerequisite for success (*Table 24*) (Porritt, 1990). The learning process is hindered by non-therapeutic communication (*Table 25*).

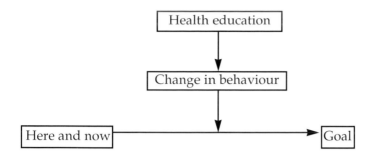

Figue 42. Education for change.

Table 24. The basic elements of therapeutic, patient-centred communication

- *Physical closeness:* the nurse indicates to the patient that she is willing to become involved.
- *Active listening:* the nurse communicates her interest in the patient non-verbally.
- *Open-ended comments:* the patient is allowed to determine the direction that the interaction should take.
- *Acknowledgement:* of the patient's comments as of value.
- *Restating/seeking clarification:* the nurse confirms the accuracy of her own appraisal of the patient's problems, at the same time demonstrating a desire to understand the problem from the patient's perspective.
- *Focusing/summarising:* helps to clarify the most important issues for both parties.
- *Mutual decision making:* deciding on goals and future actions together in a way which emphasises the patient's involvement.

Table 25. Indicators of non-therapeutic communication

- *Maintaining a distance/walking away:* the nurse suggests that she is unwilling to interact with the patient, or regards interaction as a low priority.
- *Failure to listen:* the nurse places her needs above those of the patient and demonstrates a lack of interest and concern.
- *Changing the topic:* indicates to the patient that the nurse is in control of what can and cannot be discussed, negates concept of mutuality.
- *Peremptory reassurance:* denies validity of patient's fears and feelings.
- *Being judgmental/giving advice:* by imposing her own assessment of the situation the nurse is denying the patient's rights to have opinions and make decisions

5.3   Assessment

The first stage in planning an individualised health education programme is assessment of the patient's existing knowledge, cognitive abilities, and specific problems and needs. Empathy is important. It encourages:

- More accurate understanding between the nurse and the patient.
- Greater flow of information.
- Rapid correction of misunderstandings.
- Higher levels of morale in both parties.

The nurse needs to be able to define the patient's *learning needs* and the patient's *readiness* for health education. A patient's readiness may be inhibited by physical factors, such as poorly controlled pain or disturbed sleep patterns, or psychosocial factors, such as a recent bereavement, anxiety and/or depression.

5.4   Planning

Planning a long-term education programme involves:

- Determining short, medium, and long-term learning objectives.
- Selecting the most appropriate teaching strategies for the patient and the subject matter.
- Developing ways of evaluating the effectiveness of the teaching–learning experience.

Teaching strategies might include demonstrations, use of video tapes, slides, models, books, and pamphlets. A very readable account of teaching strategies is given by Coutts and Hardy (1985). Ewles and Simnett (1992) describe ways of producing and using a variety of health promotion materials. Examples of patient information leaflets, written for alert patients and/or their carers, are given in Appendices 5.1–5.3. There is no doubt that clear *written* instructions can increase compliance with treatment, but they are no substitute for careful explanation and continuous reinforcement of the requisite self-help skills.

Successful teaching requires considerable insight on the part of the educator as to the patient's needs and capabilities, and the careful selection and use of a range of approaches appropriate to that individual. Heron (1991) describes six major categories of counselling interventions:

- *Prescriptive intervention:* seeks to *direct the behaviour* of the client.
- *Informative intervention:* seeks to *impart knowledge*, information, and meaning.
- *Confronting intervention:* seeks to *raise the client's consciousness* of some limiting attitude or behaviour.
- *Cathartic intervention:* seeks to enable the client to *discharge some pent-up emotion* such as grief, fear and anger.
- *Catalytic intervention:* seeks to elicit *self-directed learning* and *problem solving* in the client.
- *Supportive intervention:* seeks to *affirm the worth* of the client as a person.

The first three interventions are described as *authoritative* because they are rather more hierarchical, with the practitioner taking responsibility for, and on behalf of, the client. The second three are described as *facilitative*, as the practitioner is seeking to enable clients to become more autonomous. No one way is intrinsically better than another in all circumstances. The needs of the client, the nature of the client–practitioner relationship and the focus of the intervention will determine which types of intervention are likely to be of most value in a particular situation.

A more detailed discussion of teaching interventions and strategies is beyond the scope of this book. The reader is strongly advised to consult several of the texts recommended in Further Reading, and, where possible, to undertake further training in teaching and counselling skills.

5.5 Implementation and evaluation

Implementation involves putting the teaching plan into action, using non-technical language that the patient can understand, at an appropriate time and in an appropriate place.

Some of the basic principles of effective teaching are:

- To organise the material into a logical framework.
- To work from the known to the unknown.
- To give the most important information first.
- To give specific rather than general advice.
- To maximise patient involvement.
- To use a variety of teaching methods, even within the same session.
- To ensure relevance of the material to the patient's needs.
- To verify at every stage that the teaching is understood.

It is important to try to assess the extent to which the learning objectives have been achieved, by gently probing questions to test the patient's understanding of the subject and by observing whether the patient's behaviour has changed in a way which will promote health. Some of the teaching will involve physical skills training, such as the application of a compression stocking. Supervised practice will be required until the patient is, and feels, safely competent.

Many elderly and infirm patients rely on help from relatives, friends or neighbours with various activities of daily living.

Identifying who the principal carers are and including them in the teaching sessions and in care planning is of fundamental importance to the success of any teaching programme.

Further reading

Burnand, P. (1989) *Counselling Skills for Health Professionals* Chapman and
    Hall, London.
Claxton, G. (1984) *Live and Learn: An Introduction to the Psychology of Growth
    and Change in Everyday Life* Harper and Row, London.
Coutts, L.C. & Hardy, L.K. (1985) *Teaching for Health: the Nurse as Health
    Educator* Churchill Livingstone, Edinburgh.
Ewles, L. & Simnett, I. (1992) *Promoting Health: A Practical Guide* (2nd edn)
    Scutari Press, London.
Heron, J. (1991) *Helping the Client: A Creative Practical Guide* Sage
    Publications, London.
Porritt, L. (1990) *Interaction Strategies: An Introduction for Health
    Professionals* (2nd edn) Churchill Livingstone, Edinburgh.
Tschudin, V. (1991) *Counselling Skills for Nurses* (3rd edn.) Bailliere Tindall,
    London.

References

Coutts, L.C. & Hardy, L.K. (1985) *Teaching for Health: the Nurse as Health Educator*
    Churchill Livingstone, Edinburgh.
Ewles, L. & Simnett, I. (1992) Using and producing health promotion materials. In:
    Ewles, L. & Simnett, I. *Promoting Health: A Practical Guide.* (2nd edn) Scutari
    Press, London, pp. 226–242.
Heron, J. (1991) *Helping the Client: A Creative Practical Guide* Sage Publications,
    London.
Porritt, L. (1990) The challenge of listening: how to read the music of the message.
    In: Porritt, L. *Interaction Strategies: An Introduction for Health Professionals.* (2nd
    edn) Churchill Livingstone, Edinburgh, pp. 81–96.
Tschudin, V. (1991) *Counselling Skills for Nurses* (3rd edn.) Bailliere Tindall,
    London.
Weinman, J. (1982) Psychological reactions to physical illness and handicap. In:
    Weinman, J. *An Outline of Psychology as Applied to Medicine.* John Wright,
    Bristol, pp. 206–221.

Appendix 5.1
Diabetic patient information leaflet: foot care

Advice to diabetic patients on foot care
Do:

- Wash feet daily.
- Dry feet well, especially between the toes.
- Check your feet at least once a day for early signs of redness, blisters, or any other minor damage; always check between the toes and the soles of the feet (a mirror may help with this). If your vision is impaired, ask a friend to do this for you.
- Consult the doctor at once for even minor foot injuries.
- Change socks and/or stockings daily.
- Before putting shoes on, check the insides for small stones or other foreign bodies.
- Consult a chiropodist about care of toenails, calluses, and any other foot problems, and tell the chiropodist that you are diabetic.
- Have new shoes fitted by a trained fitter. Your chiropodist will advise whether or not you need special shoes, and, if so, how to obtain them.
- Avoid extremes of temperature. Use a bath thermometer to check that the water temperature does not exceed 43°C, and avoid extreme cold, as chilblains can lead to ulcers. It is useful to wear fleecy lined boots in winter.

Do not:

- Attempt your own chiropody or use chemicals to remove corns or calluses or to treat an infection.
- Wear socks or stockings with bulky seams or other potential pressure points.
- Wear shoes without socks or stockings.
- Wear anything that restricts blood circulation in the legs and feet, such as garters or tight corsets.
- Walk barefoot, especially on hot surfaces such as a sandy beach.
- Sit too close to the fire (instead, use extra socks and fleecy lined slippers to keep your feet warm).
- Put your feet on a hot water bottle.
- Soak your feet for prolonged periods.
- Smoke.

Appendix 5.2

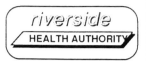

VENOUS LEG ULCERS
Helping your leg ulcer to heal

What causes leg ulcers ?

The veins in your legs are not working well - the
veins become unhealthy and congested.
Ulcers are more likely to occur - particularly if
your leg is knocked - and they take a long time to heal.

How your nurse helps....

She dresses the ulcer. She puts tight elastic bandages
on your leg. This firmly supports the unhealthy veins,
improves the circulationand encourages healing.

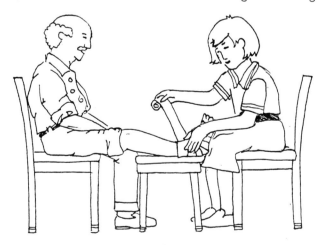

Helping your leg ulcer to heal

● You can help by............
Exercising outdoors
Go for walks. Exercise those leg muscles to clear out congestion. Get the blood pumping around!

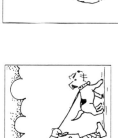

●...and indoors
Keep the blood circulating by moving your foot up and down whenever you get the chance and as often as possible.

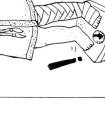

● You can help by............
...resting properly
Don't just sit down, take the load off your legs - put your feet up!

Raise your feet **higher** than your heart to help the blood circulate and speed healing.

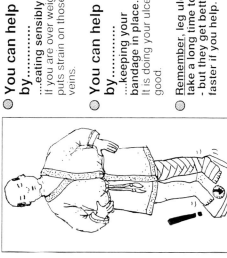

Heart

Cushions

Ankles above heart. Do **not** cross your legs.

● You can help by............
...eating sensibly
If you are over weight it puts strain on those poor veins.

● You can heal by............
...keeping your bandage in place. It is doing your ulcer good.

● Remember, leg ulcers take a long time to heal - but they get better faster if you help.

When your ulcer has gone
**Keep up the good work
(exercising/resting properly)**

◎ **Support your legs with medical elastic stockings before you get out of bed**
(Don't give your veins the chance to fill up and become congested again.)

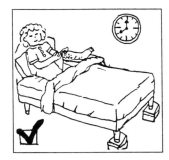

◎ **Don't toast your legs**
Help keep those veins healthy

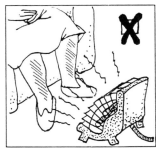

◎ **Avoid injury**
A knock could start off an ulcer again.

◎ **If you notice any sign of an ulcer starting, consult your nurse or doctor.**

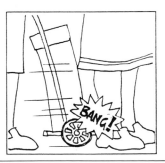

Appendix 5.3

COMPRESSION STOCKINGS

Compression stockings prevent fluid from building up and give firm support to the legs. To be effective, stockings must be **firm-fitting** and be worn **every day.**

Instructions for wearing stockings

⊚ You must put on your stockings first thing in the morning before your legs begin to swell.

⊚ Applying moisturising cream at night prevents difficulty in putting on your stockings next morning

Leg stockings

1) The basic stocking.

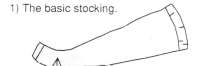

2) Turn stocking inside out up to the heel.

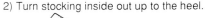
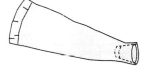

3) Place slipper over foot

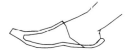

4) Pull foot of stocking over foot.

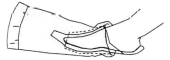

5) Gradually ease stocking up over heel and ankle.

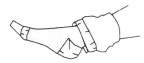

6) Ease rest of stocking a bit at a time up the leg. Do not pull from the top.

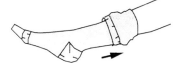

7) Pull out slipper liner through opening at toes.

8) If this is a knee-length stocking, the top should reach the crease behind the knee - **no further.**

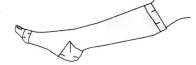

It should fit smoothly along the leg. There should be no creases or wrinkles

Question : Should I remove my stocking if I experience aching or tightness in my leg ?

Answer : No, this is probably due to a period of inactivity and a build-up of fluid in the leg. Try walking around or exercising the leg as follows...

slowly and firmly point foot towards floor, then bring back as far as it will go.
repeat 10 times.

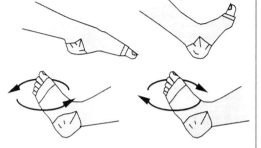

slowly and firmly rotate feet, making circular movements with pointed toes. First clockwise, then anticlockwise.
repeat 10 times.

It is important to raise the legs as often as possible

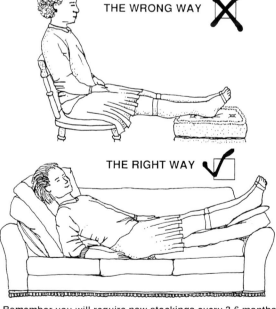

THE WRONG WAY

THE RIGHT WAY

Remember you will require new stockings every 3-6 months or when hosiery loses its firmness

6. Quality assurance

6.0 Introduction

In 1989, the Government published a White Paper called 'Working for Patients' (Department of Health, 1989). This was incorporated by Parliament into the 1990 NHS and Community Care Act. It has led to radical changes in the way that the NHS is organised and financed.

The aim of the changes, first announced in 'Working for Patients', is to raise the *quality* of health care, delivered by all GP practices and hospitals, to that of the best. The implication, borne out by a number of national clinical and financial audit studies, is that the quality and cost of services offered to patients varies considerably between hospitals and community units, and at the individual practitioner level. At the same time patients' *expectations* of the health service are increasing.

Health care professionals are being actively encouraged by the Royal Colleges and by Health Services Management to *review their practice systematically and critically*. This is audit. Recognition of the benefits of clinical audit is growing within the professions themselves, but there is still some confusion about fundamental concepts relating to quality assurance in health care, and this is not helped by the variety of definitions of some very commonly used terms.

This chapter begins by exploring the concept of quality, and the benefits of a high quality service from the perspective of the patient, the health care professional and management. The meaning of terms such as 'quality assurance', 'quality control', 'quality systems', 'standard setting' and 'audit' will be explained before looking in more detail at how to audit a service. The chapter ends by outlining some key professional issues for the future.

A particularly fine example of the application of these principles to the setting up of community leg ulcer clinics is given in Chapter 7. This example shows how quality assurance can be built in to every stage of reorganising and implementing an integrated service.

6.1   What is quality?

Ovretveit defines quality in relation to the health services as:

'Fully meeting the needs of those who need the service most, at the lowest cost to the organisation, within limits and directives set by higher authorities and purchasers.'

Ovretveit (1992), p. 2.

This definition of quality combines the dimensions of quality described by Shaw (1986) (*Table 26*), namely: appropriateness, effectiveness, acceptability, accessibility, and efficiency, with the legal, ethical and contractual requirements of 'higher authorities', such as the Government, professional bodies and the purchasers of services.

Providing a quality service therefore involves:

- Meeting or exceeding the expectations of customers.
- Meeting or exceeding professionally agreed standards.
- Improving efficiency and reducing costs.

The 'customer' may be an individual patient, his or her family, or the community to be served.

The definition implies that, while the customer's view is of central importance, patients are not competent to judge the level of *technical* excellence of their care, which is the role of health care professionals through *peer review*. The purchaser's role is to assess the health needs of the *populations* that they serve, to place contracts with providers of services to meet these needs, and to get value for money.

There will inevitably, at times, be a conflict of interest between customer defined quality, professionally defined quality and management's definition of quality. Any *quality system* needs to incorporate mechanisms for dealing with this conflict. A quality system encompasses the organisational structure, responsibilities, procedures, processes and resources for implementing quality management (British Standards Institute, 1987).

Table 26. Dimensions of quality of health care (based on Shaw, 1986)

- *Appropriateness* Meeting the actual needs of individuals, families and communities
- *Effectiveness* Achieving the intended benefit
- *Acceptability* Satisfying patient's reasonable expectations
- *Continuity* Of care and care provider(s)
- *Accessibility* Availability not unduly restricted by time, distance or finance
- *Efficiency* Maximising outcomes with the available resources

6.2 Why adopt a quality approach?

The demand for, and the cost of, health care in the western world is rising at such an alarming rate that it is becoming a very political issue in some countries.

In the USA, health care costs rose by $80 billion between 1991 and 1992 to $817 billion, or 14% of the gross national product (Berwick, 1992). Costs are rising in the UK too, although less steeply.

The quickest way for any 'firm' to go out of business is to provide a high quality service without due regard to cost. In a publicly financed health service, where demand is outstripping supply, there need to be incentives to increase efficient use of resources (Davies, 1992). Improving the quality of a service can not only *reduce needless patient suffering* but can also reduce costs, allowing resources to be reallocated to others in need. It can do this directly by:

- Increasing the appropriateness of care and reducing unnecessary tests and procedures.
- Reducing avoidable complications and prolonged treatment times.
- Reducing wastage of materials.
- Reducing costs of dealing with complaints.
- Reducing claims for negligence.
- Increasing throughput, where the money follows the patient.

Furthermore, a high quality service is more likely to retain a motivated, well trained work force, who are committed to the organisation's aims and objectives. Delivering high quality care is less frustrating and more satisfying for staff, and leads to higher morale, better interdisciplinary cooperation, and therefore better standards of patient care.

The ethical and professional requirements always to act in the client's best interests are self evident, and the cornerstone of healthcare professionals' codes of professional conduct.

The value of adopting a *research based approach to practice*, in the management of leg ulcers, was described in Chapter 1. Dramatic improvements in healing rates, and in the patients' quality of life, can be achieved, while at the same time providing a cost effective service.

Adopting a quality approach means a better service for patients, families and communities.

6.3 Quality assurance and leg ulcer care

The British Standards Institute's definition of *quality assurance* is:

> 'A management system designed to give the maximum confidence that a given acceptable level of quality of service is being achieved with a minimum of total expenditure.'
>
> British Standards Institute (1987)

Ovretveit defines it as:

> 'All activities undertaken to predict and prevent poor quality'
>
> Ovretveit (1992) p. 164

Quality control is a part of quality assurance and is:

> 'The process through which we measure actual quality performance, compare it with a standard and act on the difference'
>
> Juran and Gryna (1980)

Clinical audit contributes to quality assurance, and involves a cycle of activities (*Figure 43*). The emphasis should be on closing the audit loop; that is, rectifying any deficiencies identified, and repeating the exercise to see whether in fact anything has changed.

Leg ulcer care lends itself to audit because:

- Large numbers of patients in hospital and the community have a leg ulcer at some point in their lives (Section 1.1).
- There is a high risk of the ulcer becoming intractable with prolonged, inappropriate care (Section 1.4).
- Leg ulcers cause considerable patient suffering and adversely affect many aspects of quality of life (Section 1.6).
- Leg ulcers cost the NHS a considerable amount of money (Section 1.5).
- Most leg ulcers heal rapidly with appropriate care (Section 1.4).

The next question is what to audit? Some factors to consider are given in *Figure 44*. The focus should be on measuring outcomes such as:

- Healing rates.
- Quality of life, at various points during and after treatment.
- Patient satisfaction with service.
- Patient understanding of, and compliance with, self-help advice to promote healing and prevent recurrence.

It is also very important to audit the *process* of care, as a high quality process should lead to the optimal outcome for the individual. Morison (1992a) described how the process of wound care was audited in a Community Unit in Scotland. Sixty-nine Community Nurses (97% of such

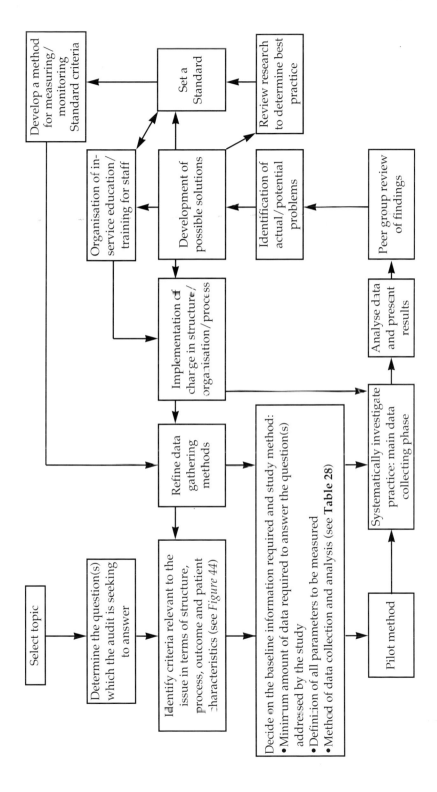

Figure 43. The audit process (modified from Morison, 1991).

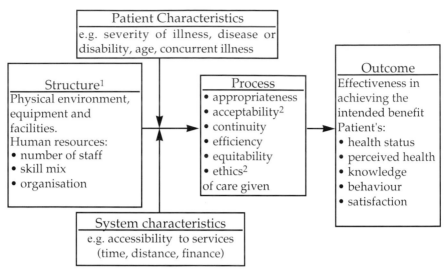

Figure 44. What to audit? Some factors to consider when developing a programme to measure the quality of care (based on Donabedian, 1969; Shaw, 1986; Hopkins, 1990).

Notes: [1] *Simply determines the potential for, or constraints against, the delivery of high quality care.*

[2] *Ultimately a social construct, influenced by social values.*

nurses at work at the time of the study) kept a structured diary for one week, in which they recorded the nature of each wound, how long the patient had been treated (*Figure 1*), the number and duration of visits in a week (*Table 3*), the wound care products used, and any additional activities undertaken by the nurse at each visit. In a separate questionnaire, the staff were asked about the sources of information they used concerning wound care products. Most nurses turned to another nursing colleague as the first choice for information and advice. Nurses were asked about their continuing education experiences and perceived needs in relation to wound care.

Feedback of the results of the audit gave staff considerable insights into their own practice. It highlighted some of the problems of wound dressing selection (*Table 27*) and the need for a local formulary, which has since been developed. It also identified the need for more educational material. One of the many positive outcomes from this study was the development of a computer assisted learning package to facilitate distance learning in relation to the assessment and management of leg ulcers. Doppler ultrasound equipment was bought to aid patient assessment. This was purchased using money raised from a clinical bandage trial. The trial in itself raised awareness of good assessment and management principles. The need for a *standard* on wound assessment in the community was also identified, and a standard was developed in one community unit.

What is a standard? A standard is a professionally agreed level of performance which is desirable, achievable, observable and measurable.

Measures by which the achievement of a standard can be assessed are:

- *Structure criteria* The resources necessary e.g. manpower, skill mix, equipment, policies and procedures.
- *Process criteria* The actions taken by staff to achieve the desired outcome.
- *Outcome criteria* The desired effect of the care process, e.g. patient health status, level of knowledge, skills acquisition, behaviour, and satisfaction with care.

Table 27. The problems of wound dressing selection

- There is a bewildering variety of dressings from which to choose
- Many products which look alike have different physical and chemical properties
- Different manufacturers recommend different types of products for the same problem
- Therapeutic traditions may make it difficult to introduce 'new generation' products
- There is a blurring of responsibility between health care professionals in relation to prescribing
- Health economics in relation to wound care are complex – products with a higher unit cost may in fact be very cost effective
- New products and types of product are appearing on the market every month
- Many wound dressings used in hospital are not available in the community
- There are restrictions in the sizes of many dressings available in the community

The standard setting cycle (*Figure 45*) is a form of audit in which the minimum standard to be achieved or exceeded is made very explicit for a particular care group (the group of patients to whom the standard applies). More details of the RCN's *Dynamic Standard Setting System* are given in Royal College of Nursing (1990).

Success in closing the standard setting loop (*Figure 45*) and improving patient care depends upon:

- Ownership of the standard by the staff themselves (Morison, 1992b).
- Management's commitment to rectifying any deficiencies found.
- A reliable and valid method of data collection (*Figure 46*).

Some of the most commonly used methods of measuring are listed in *Table 28*. It is very important to obtain professional advice on the method and design of questionnaires and other data collecting tools. For larger studies, the statistician's advice should be sought on sample size and methods of data analysis *before* data collection begins.

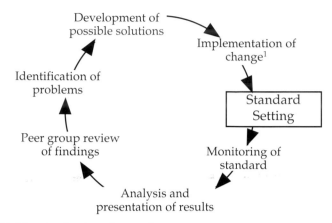

Figure 45. The standard setting cycle.
[1] *Implementation of change may include modification of the standard.*

Piloting the method is essential, to ensure:

- That it results in the collection of useful, unambiguous data.
- That the people collecting the data understand the definitions of terms.
- That the method is practicable.

Issues of *confidentiality and data protection* must be addressed at the outset.

Creating a climate of enquiry is of paramount importance. Initial resistance to being involved in audit is both natural and understandable (*Table 29*). One definition of audit is 'a calling to account', which has many negative connotations. People may feel threatened by audit, both personally and professionally, which is why it is so important from the outset to develop an atmosphere of mutual support and trust, address the issues of data confidentiality and spend time explaining, to all those involved, the nature and purpose of the audit (Morison, 1992b). It is important to emphasise that audit is not just about identifying problems. Good practice is also highlighted. It is very satisfying for staff to know when they are achieving the high standards that they are setting for themselves, and that they can indeed assure the 'customer' of a specified degree of excellence in the service.

Ideally, the staff themselves should collectively decide the priorities for local audit studies, and should be involved in planning the study as well as peer review of the results.

Table 28. Some commonly used methods of measuring

- Patient satisfaction questionnaires.
- Questionnaires to staff.
- Audit of documentation.
- Direct observation of practice.
- Structured diaries recording practice.
- Structured interviews with patients.
- Structured interviews with staff.

Table 29. Reasons for resistance to clinical audit

- Personal threat.
- Fear of uses to which data might be put by management.
- Time constraints.
- Lack of belief in potential benefits.

Recognising resistance:

- Lip Service.
- Lethargy.
- Aggression.
- Lack of Continuity.

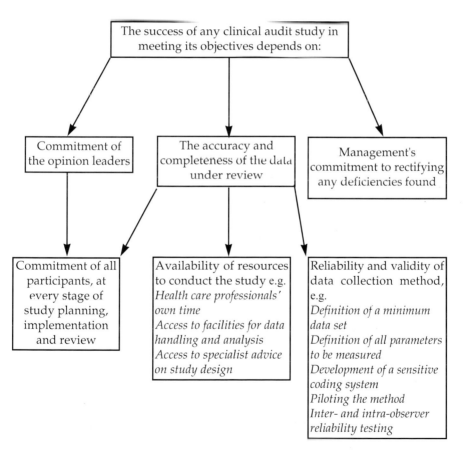

Figure 46. Requirements for a successful outcome to a clinical audit study.

In reality, there can be a considerable time lag before the majority of people take up a new innovation (Stocking, 1992), and clinical audit is still regarded by some people as new. The commitment of opinion leaders can make all the difference to the success of an audit study. Opinion leaders can help to maintain the impetus during the data collecting phase, but they are also crucial in ensuring that any new practice guidelines introduced as a result of the study are carried out (Lomas *et al.*, 1991).

6.4   The way forward

Clinical audit can be done on many levels. It is possible to audit:

- A *procedure*, such as aseptic wound dressing technique, which is specified in detail in the Unit's procedure manual.
- A *standard*, developed by staff, relating to a particular topic such as wound assessment or pain control.
- An *episode of care*, such as a planned skin graft.

It is also possible to audit a whole service (Chapter 7).

The challenge is to capture accurate, useful data on all patients in an ongoing way, or to sample the activity to be audited systematically, in a way that ensures that the sample is representative of the population as a whole.

There are very few aspects of health care which involve only one professional group, yet uniprofessional audit studies are still the most common. There is a move towards multidisciplinary clinical audit, which is particularly appropriate in the case of the management of patients with leg ulcers. Experiments in collaborative care planning (Finnegan, 1991) are evolving to include, in many cases, joint care planning, a single set of documentation used by all health care professionals, and collectively agreed goals and shared audit processes. Patient satisfaction questionnaires may be 'grafted on' to gain an insight into the customer's perspective. It is very rare, however, to find an integrated study which combines the patients', the health care professionals', and management's perspectives of quality (Section 6.1), by looking at patient satisfaction, the attainment of professionally agreed standards of clinical practice, and value for money.

Once health care professionals have become more familiar with standard setting and methods of measuring quality, it may then be possible to introduce a total quality management (TQM) approach, which helps to overcome the rather skewed perspective gained from looking at the clinical aspects of care alone.

***Total Quality Management* is an approach to creating and maintaining a system of improvement in a complex organisation.**

TQM goes beyond the processes and practices of quality assurance and quality control. It involves changing the culture of the organisation, requiring all staff at all levels to be involved in the process of quality improvement. The characteristics and philosophy of TQM are summarised in *Table 30*.

Table 30. The characteristics and philosophy of TQM.

TQM is characterised by:

- The declared intention to strive for *continuous improvement*; this means exceeding targets, not just meeting them.
- A definition of quality which focuses on meeting the needs of the *customer* and meeting or exceeding customer expectations.
- A total commitment to quality by top management.
- Action oriented measurement systems, and translating good ideas originating from staff into action.
- An acknowledgement of the interdependency of all staff and the encouragement of collaborative practices.
- Investment in staff development.
- The recognition that when things go wrong the problem is most likely to be due to a failure or fault in a process or in systems rather than to be the fault of individuals. The premise is that most people want to do a good job (unless they have been totally demoralised and alienated by management, which does indeed indicate faulty processes). The solution lies in identifying the faults in processes and correcting them rather than blaming individuals.
- Systematic elimination of waste, duplication of effort and the use of unnecessary or unproven practices.

It is impossible to introduce TQM unless there is a *quality system* in place (Section 6.1). The introduction of a quality approach, whether or not this is based on the philosophy of total quality management, requires the development of: a quality policy, an overall quality strategy, and specific quality programmes.

A quality policy is a general guide outlining the organisation's philosophy and how quality activities will be organised and carried out. *Quality programmes* are more short term plans to achieve certain specific strategy objectives within a given time frame. An overall *quality strategy* is the general long-term plan for introducing and improving service quality, and for changing the orientation of the organisation's culture to the pursuit of excellence through a number of quality programmes.

Above all, introducing a quality approach requires *facilitative leadership* (Morison, 1992b), with the leader acting as change agent who:

- Encourages staff participation and ownership.
- Explains *and demonstrates* the benefits of a quality approach.
- Removes any perceived threats to staff members' status, responsibility, values, pay and working conditions.
- Improves channels and mechanisms for communication.
- Identifies staff development needs and organises relevant education and training.
- Identifies and wins over the enthusiasts and opinion leaders.

Quality is a philosophy: introducing a quality approach involves changing the hearts and minds of all those involved in patient care, whether directly or indirectly, so that all are committed to striving for continuous improvement in the service.

An extensive Further Reading list has been included to help the reader to explore the topic of quality assurance in more depth. It includes extensive references to a variety of methods of measurement of health status and quality of life.

Further reading

Quality Assurance in the NHS

Kitson, A. & Harvey, G. (1991) *Bibliography of Nursing Quality Assurance and Standards of Care* Scutari Press, Harrow.

Koch, H. (1991) *Total Quality Management in Health Care* Longman.

Morison, M.J. (1992) Promoting the motivation to change: the role of facilitative leadership in quality assurance. *Professional Nurse* **August**, 715–718.

Ovretveit, J. (1992) *Health Service Quality: An Introduction to Quality Methods for Health Services* Blackwell Scientific Publications, Oxford.

Pearson, A. (ed) (1987) *Nursing Quality Measurement: Quality Assurance Methods for Peer Review* John Wiley, Chichester.

Redfern, S.J. & Norman, I.J. (1990) Measuring the quality of nursing care: a consideration of differing approaches. *J Adv Nurs* **15**, 1260–1271.

Royal College of Nursing (1990) *Standards of Care Project. Quality Patient Care: The Dynamic Standard Setting System* RCN, London.

Wright, C. & Whittington, D. (1992) *Quality Assurance: An Introduction for Health Care Professionals* Churchill Livingstone, Edinburgh.

Quality Assurance and Wound Care

Balc, S. (1989) Cost effective wound management in the community. *Professional Nurse* **12**, 598–601.

Griffey, M. (1992) Reach for the highest standard: comparison of leg ulcer management in two practices. *Professional Nurse* **8(3)**, 189–192.

Morison, M.J. (1992) Quality assurance and wound care in the community. *Ostomy/Wound Management* **38(8)**, 38–44.

Measuring Health Status and Quality of Life

Bardsley, M. & Coles, J. (1992) Practical experiences in auditing patient outcomes. *Quality in Health Care* **1**, 124–130.

Bowling, A. (1991) *Measuring Health: A Review of Quality of Life Measuring Scales* Oxford University Press, Milton Keynes.

Cox, D., Fitzpatrick, R., Fletcher, A., Gore, S., Spiegelhalter, D. & Jones, D. (1992) Quality of life assessment: can we keep it simple? *Journal of the Royal Statistical Society Series A* **155**, 353–393.

Hopkins, A. (ed) (1992) *Measures of the Quality of Life: and the uses to which such measures may be put* Royal College of Physicians, London.

McDowell, I. & Newell, C. (1987) *Measuring Health: A Guide to Rating Scales and Questionnaires* Oxford University Press, Oxford.

Wilkin, D., Hallam, L. & Doggett, M. (1992) *Measures of Need and Outcome for Primary Health Care* Oxford University Press, Oxford.

References

Berwick, D.M. (1992) Heal thyself or heal thy system: can doctors help to improve medical care? *Quality in Health Care* **1 (Supplement)**, S2–S8.

British Standards Institute (1987) *Quality Systems Part 1: Specification for Design/development, Production, Installation and Servicing (BSI 5750)* British Standards Institute, Milton Keynes.

Davies, H. (1992) Role of the Audit Commission. *Quality in Health Care* **1 (Supplement)**, S36–S39.

Department of Health (1989) *Working for Patients* HMSO, London.

Donabedian, A. (1969) Some issues in evaluating the quality of nursing care. *Am J Public Health* **39(10)**, 1833–1836.

Finnegan, E. (1991) *Collaborative Care Planning: A Natural Catalyst for Change* Resource Management Support Unit, West Midlands Health Region, Birmingham.

Hopkins, A. (1990) *Measuring Quality of Medical Care* Royal College of Physicians, London.

Juran, J.M. & Gryna, F.M. (1980) *Quality Planning and Analysis* McGraw–Hill, New Delhi.

Lomas, J., Enkin, M., Anderson, G.M., Hannah, W.J., Vayda, E. & Singer, J. (1991) Opinion leaders vs audit and feedback to implement practice guidelines. *JAMA* **265 (17)**, 2202–2207.

Morison, M.J. (1991) The Stirling model of nursing audit. *Professional Nurse* **6 (7)**, Wallchart.

Morison, M.J. (1992a) Quality assurance and wound care in the community. *Ostomy/Wound Management* **38(8)**, 38–44.

Morison, M.J. (1992b) Promoting the motivation to change: the role of facilitative leadership in quality assurance. *Professional Nurse* **August**, 715–718.

Ovretveit, J. (1992) *Health Service Quality: An Introduction to Quality Methods for Health Services* Blackwell Scientific Publications, Oxford.

Royal College of Nursing, (1990) *Standards of Care Project. Quality Patient Care: The Dynamic Standard Setting System* RCN, London.

Shaw, C.D. (1986) *Introducing Quality Assurance. Paper No. 64* Kings Fund, London,

Stocking, B. (1992) Promoting change in clinical care. *Quality in Health Care* **1**, 56–60.

7. Providing a service

7.0 Introduction

The National Health Service is undergoing considerable change, with the emphasis shifting to community care.

The majority of patients with leg ulcers have traditionally been cared for in the community (Section 1.3). Having appreciated the considerable resources involved in caring for this patient group, an increasing number of health authorities is seeking to develop district-wide leg ulcer services. There is a great deal of scope for districts to develop innovative services that meet the needs of the local population, and use the expertise available in both the acute and community services.

Recent research has indicated that by implementing research based practice within a rationalised service, the healing rates of venous ulcers can be dramatically improved (Section 1.4). For this to be achieved, there needs to be a shift away from 'maintaining' the current situation, where ulcers remain unhealed for long periods, to services where effective treatment results in rapid ulcer healing, improved quality of life for patients, and cost-effective care.

This chapter highlights the factors to consider when establishing a service (*Table 31*), and describes how an integrated leg ulcer service was established and evaluated at Riverside.

7.1 The Riverside Community Leg Ulcer Project

The Riverside Community Leg Ulcer Project took a fresh approach to the organisation of the management of leg ulceration within the community. A network of community leg ulcer clinics was set up in health centres and clinics throughout the district. Links were established with the Vascular Surgical Service at Charing Cross Hospital providing an integrated service for all patients with leg ulcers in the district (*Figures 47, 48*).

7.1.1 Assessing the problem

Before the clinics were opened, a control audit was carried out to examine current practice and efficacy of treatment. This showed that although many products were used to treat leg ulcers, adequate compression was rarely used. The audit was carried out within one health centre over an 18 week period. Nurses recorded all visits to leg ulcer patients, and noted

Table 31. Factors to consider when establishing a service

- The size of the problem

  Establish the size of the problem within an area: what is the prevalence of ulceration, who is treating leg ulcers and where? The true scale of the problem may not be immediately apparent, with patients presenting from a number of sources.

- Support and resources

  To succeed the service will need to be well-supported and resourced by management. Managers will need evidence to support proposed improvements in practice. This evidence can come from a critical review of published research and from auditing current services (Chapter 6).

- Multidisciplinary involvement

  To ensure that the professional expertise of all relevant disciplines is available when appropriate to all patients.

- Integration

  Integration of acute and community services provides the most effective service for patients.

- Coordination

  A key professional should be responsible for monitoring the service, and ensuring that new research is implemented in clinical practice.

- Research-based protocols

  The service should deliver care, firmly grounded in best practice as identified from the latest research, to all leg ulcer patients.

- Training

  A comprehensive and on-going training programme will need to be developed which reflects the needs of the nurse practitioner.

- Accessibility

  The service should be flexible in its organisation and allow easy access for patients seeking treatment.

- Transport

  A cost-effective, reliable transport system will need to be developed if patients are to be brought to a clinic.

- Evaluation

  The service will require regular evaluation to ensure standards are maintained and health outcomes met.

when they healed. Fifty-one patients were treated, in a total of 865 home visits. The healing rate study showed that only 22% of ulcers were healed within 12 weeks using conventional methods (*Table 1*). The cost of care within the district was established. The major cost was in district nursing time, with Riverside district nurses spending 25% of their time caring for leg ulcer patients (Section 1.5).

7.1.2 Planning the service

The Riverside Leg Ulcer Service involved integrating acute and community services, and was planned to meet the needs of the surrounding community. This involved close cooperation and consultation with all professionals, and establishing links with the

121

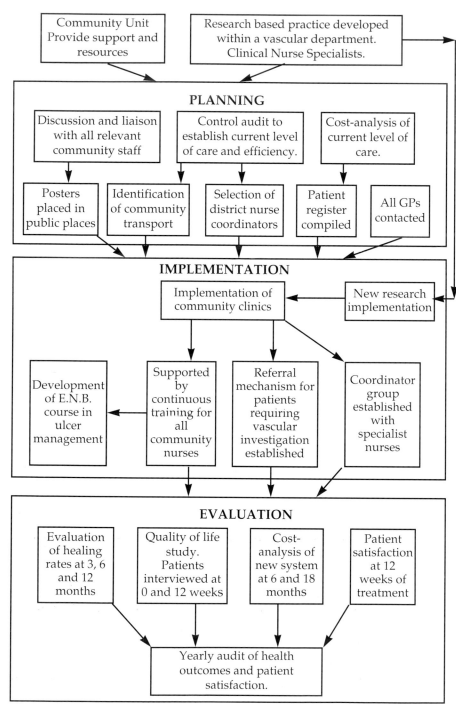

Figure 47 Development programme for Community Ulcer Clinics linked to a Vascular Surgical Service in Riverside Health Authority.

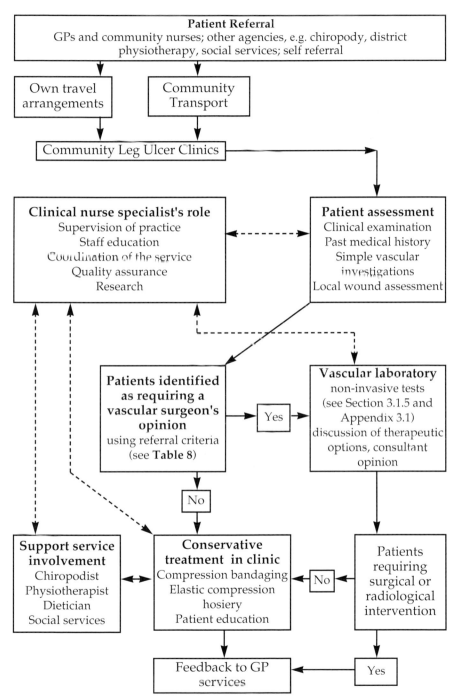

Figure 48. The relationship between Community Clinics, the vascular surgical service and other supporting agencies – common patient referral and treatment pathways.

network of support services available in both the hospital and community. Two district nurses from each clinic were nominated as coordinators, thus ensuring the smooth running of the clinics. Community management identified resources to purchase new equipment, such as portable Doppler ultrasound and the bandages used to apply compression. Three of the bandages used were not available on prescription. This proved a considerable burden at a time of great economic restraint.

Providing a reliable, cost-effective community transport system was crucial to the success of the project. An adapted ambulance was purchased, and a driver recruited. This enabled even very immobile wheelchair patients to be brought to the clinic. Referral criteria were developed in consultation with the vascular unit, to identify patients requiring further investigation and treatment at hospital. These patients were referred by the nurse specialist for full investigation and consultant opinion. The majority of patients remained in the community to receive their treatment.

7.1.3 Implementation of the service

Clinics were opened at three-monthly intervals to allow for a programme of in-service training. Staff rotated through the clinics and received training from the specialist nurses. The aim of training was to equip the community nurses caring for leg ulcer patients with the knowledge and skills to use the new research-based methods.

Protocols were implemented for the management of venous ulcers and ulcers of other aetiologies.

Integration of the Service was enhanced by a coordinator group, which met regularly with the specialist nurses. This provided a focus for discussion and training.

The community transport system was able to bring 12 patients to each of the six community clinics. Only 11% of the patients within the district were too frail or immobile to attend the clinic, and those were assessed and treated by the district nurse at home.

7.1.4 Patient referral

Of the 475 patients attending the ulcer clinics in the 2-year study period, only 46% had been cared for previously by district nurses. Surprisingly, 25% of patients self-referred, and were not known to health professionals. This clearly indicated the existence of a hitherto unmet need in the community, and it is likely that this group of patients would develop chronic, intractable ulceration requiring a high level of care at a later date. The nature of patients' ulcers were as follows:

- 475 patients with 550 leg ulcers.
- 17% bilateral ulceration.
- 83% unilateral ulceration.
- 10% (56) significant arterial disease (resting pressure index 0.5–0.8).
- 1% (8) rheumatoid arthritis.
- 1% (6) diabetic foot ulceration.
- 4 skin cancers.

7.1.5   Evaluating patient outcomes and cost effectiveness

In evaluating the project the following aspects were considered:

- *Changes in ulcer healing rates* Ulcer healing rates rose within 12 weeks of a clinic opening to 55% at 12 weeks, compared to 22% healed at 12 weeks in the control unit. The healing rates continued to rise as the clinics developed. After 6–9 months, 78% were healed at 12 weeks, and after 12–15 months, 86% at 12 weeks (Table 1). This improvement is probably a consequence of earlier referral of less chronic ulcers as the Service became established.
- *Identifying factors that delay ulcer healing* It was important to identify factors that delayed venous ulcer healing. Prolonged ulcer duration, large ulcer size, reduced mobility and limb mobility were all found to significantly delay healing (Table 2). It may be possible to influence those factors by providing earlier, effective treatment. Reduced mobility may be a consequence of ulceration rather than a cause.
- *Changes in quality of life before and after treatment* Little has been known of the impact of leg ulceration on patients' lives. The Riverside study showed that by healing the patient's ulcer there was an improvement in the patient's quality of life. A symptom rating test was performed prior to, and after 12, weeks of treatment. This showed significant reductions in levels of depression, anxiety, hostility and interference with daily and social activities. This was shown to be related to the ulcer healing, as only anxiety was reduced in patients whose ulcer failed to heal. Over 75% of patients suffered with various degrees of pain at their first visit; this was reduced significantly by 12 weeks, and is a factor that has not been previously associated with venous ulceration (Section 1.6).
- *Establishing the cost-effectiveness of the Service* The Riverside project was shown to reduce the cost of leg ulcer treatment within the district, although the community service was providing treatment for significantly more patients. The Service was transformed from a 'maintenance' service to a programme with benefits for patients, staff and managers and demonstrable improvements in health outcomes (Sections 1.4 and 1.5).
- *Assessing patient satisfaction* An important aspect in evaluating any service is to establish the patient's view of the service offered. In the Riverside study, patients completed a questionnaire after 12 weeks of treatment. This indicated a high level of satisfaction with the service, and a surprisingly high level of compliance with treatment.

Further guidance on quality assurance and clinical audit is given in Chapter 6.

7.1.6   Evaluating the training programme for nurses

Karn and Moffatt (1994) describe how, as a result of the Riverside Community Leg Ulcer Project, the specific educational needs of nurses, relating to leg ulcer management were identified, and how a specific educational strategy was devised to meet these needs.

Providing a comprehensive training programme for community nurses occupied a high proportion of specialist nurse time. A survey of district nurses in Riverside found that 96% wished for a recognised course in leg ulcer management. Having identified the key areas of development, an English National Board course in ulcer management was established in conjunction with the Riverside College of Health Studies.

The Riverside study is one example of innovation: using a new approach to an old problem. Continued support and commitment are required to maintain the level of service, which should be regularly evaluated.

Development of leg ulcer services could lead to a reduction of suffering for many thousands of patients.

Further Reading

Carnall, C. (1991) *Managing Change: Self Development for Managers* Routledge, London

Handy, C. (1993) *Understanding Organisations* Penguin, London

Leigh, A. (1988) *Effective Change – Twenty Ways to Make it Happen* IPM Publications, Wimbledon.

Moss-Kanter. R, (1983) *The Change Masters* Unwin Paperbacks

Plant, R. (1987) *Managing Change and Making it Stick* Fontana (an imprint of Harper Collins Publishers), London

Scott, C.D. & Jaffe, D.T. (1990) *Managing Organisational Change* Kogan Page, London

References

Karn, E.A. & Moffatt, C.J. (1994) Developments in the management of leg ulcers: an educational response. *Professional Nurse (in press)*.

Index